Green Smoothie Retreat

Green Smoothie Retreat

A 7-Day Plan to Detox and Revitalize at Home

VICTORIA BOUTENKO

North Atlantic Books
Berkeley, California

North Atlantic Books
P.O. Box 12327
Berkeley, California 94712

Cover photo © iStockphoto.com/IngredientsPhoto
Cover and book design by Claudia Smelser
Printed in the United States of America

Green Smoothie Retreat: A 7-Day Plan to Detox and Revitalize at Home is sponsored and published by the Society for the Study of Native Arts and Sciences (dba North Atlantic Books), an educational nonprofit based in Berkeley, California, that collaborates with partners to develop cross-cultural perspectives, nurture holistic views of art, science, the humanities, and healing, and seed personal and global transformation by publishing work on the relationship of body, spirit, and nature.

North Atlantic Books' publications are available through most bookstores. For further information, visit our website at www.northatlanticbooks.com or call 800–733–3000.

Library of Congress Cataloging-in-Publication Data
    Boutenko, Victoria.
    Green smoothie retreat: a 7-day plan to detox and revitalize at home / Victoria Boutenko.
       pages   cm
    Summary: "Health and Fitness: Nutrition; Smoothies (Beverages); Cookery (Greens)" —Provided by publisher.
    Includes bibliographical references and index.
    ISBN 978-1-58394-860-6 (paperback)—ISBN 978-1-58394-861-3 (ebook)
    1. Nutrition. 2. Smoothies (Beverages) 3. Cooking (Greens) I. Title.
    RA784.B6814 2014
    613.2—dc23
                                                                        2014013475

1   2   3   4   5   6   7   8   UNITED   19   18   17   16   15
Printed on recycled paper

CONTENTS

AUTHOR'S NOTE

Have you ever been to a healing retreat? Were you fortunate to spend several days in a peaceful sanctuary where you were only resting and healing? The participants of a retreat usually live in comfortable rooms in a pleasant environment. They communicate only with a group of like-minded people. They consume special food, participate in workshops, and partake in restorative procedures. Such retreats help people to set a number of healthy habits—such as going to bed early, eating healthier, giving up coffee, and exercising—along with learning some healthy recipes.

My family has organized a variety of healing retreats since the year 2000, and we know firsthand that it can be rather expensive. For example, we must find an appropriate venue located in a clean environment but close to the airport or railway station so that participants don't have to rent a car. The facility needs to have a certified kitchen with a walk-in cooler and be suitable for the preparation of large quantities of produce. All of these factors add to the price, thus making such a retreat unreachable for many people. However, most people are even less likely to adopt a new lifestyle while going about their daily lives. I have been teaching natural health for almost twenty years and have noticed how difficult it is for people to start a new way of living without proper preparation.

At the same time, it is possible to organize your own retreat if you know how. In this book I describe in detail what you need to know to succeed with your own healing retreat. I have chosen a green smoothie retreat because such retreats have been particularly effective in my own practice. I present recommendations, nutritional facts, and recipes for a seven-day green smoothie retreat; this way, the book can be used both by those who would like to go on a green smoothie cleanse and those who would like to include more green smoothies in their everyday lives.

From 2008 through 2013, I conducted nineteen weeklong green smoothie retreats. Most of the information in this book comes from my observations of over a thousand participants at my retreats.

PART ONE

A Guide to Your Own Retreat

ONE

CRITICAL THINKING

To find yourself, think for yourself.
—SOCRATES

Without the ability for critical thinking you have a lot fewer chances to enjoy vibrant health. Of course, you need advice and assistance from medical professionals once in a while, but I would like to emphasize that it is *you* who needs to consciously participate in making the key decisions concerning *your* health because your well-being is among your highest priorities in life. For example, when buying a car, you would never let a car salesman decide for you which car you should buy. I imagine that, if car dealers had the power to decide for their customers, we would all be driving Porsches and Lamborghinis while sinking deeply in debt. Instead, when you decide to buy a car, you first gather detailed information about prospective vehicles and only then make your choice. If you happen to buy the wrong car, though you may encounter problems, overall such a decision is not fatal because you can always replace that car with another, more suitable vehicle.

However, you cannot buy another life or another body. Your life is unique and therefore priceless, and your health is precious. Your health is yours and no one else's. Therefore, *you* are in charge of your precious health, and you would greatly benefit from understanding the main principles of human health before agreeing to any particular health treatment.

Most people now have cameras in their phones, but only photographers who understand the physical laws of reflection and optics are able to create photographic masterpieces. Similarly, a basic understanding of the principles of natural healing enables each person to significantly improve his or her health. I encourage you to do your homework and read in this book and others about the underlying principles of healing your beautiful body so that you can take better care of your health and live a longer and healthier life.

In order to grasp these principles, critical thinking is essential. Otherwise, it would be hard to understand the true cause of so-called degenerative diseases. As a result, you may start treating the symptoms of the illness instead. For example, you may start taking aspirin every time you have a headache, a fever, or another symptom. However, if you apply critical thinking, you may realize that the headache cannot be caused by an aspirin deficiency, but that it is a result of some disruption of natural processes in your body. Nevertheless, every fifth American reported taking aspirin every day in 2006.[1] Without a clear understanding of human bodily functions, it may appear natural to take lots of pills but seem abnormal, for example, to connect diabetes to a lack of workouts or skin rashes to the process of detoxing. By studying a natural approach to health, you can start understanding that only the elimination of the cause can ensure true healing of any degenerative disease. Later in this book we will talk about the two main reasons for the majority of health problems.

Nowadays, critical thinking has become many times more vital than in previous times. Two or three hundred years ago most foods were natural and safe to eat. Our ancestors only had to worry about their food's cleanliness and freshness. Of course, there were times of

---

[1] Anita Soni, *Statistical Brief #179: Aspirin Use among the Adult U.S. Noninstitutionalized Population, with and without Indicators of Heart Disease* (Rockville: Agency for Healthcare Research and Quality, 2005), 1, http://meps.ahrq.gov/mepsweb/data_files/publications /st179/stat179.pdf.

food shortages, but, in general, eating was not associated with a wide range of unsolvable health problems such as those we face today. The words "pesticides," "bovine hormones," "genetically modified," "irradiated," "synthetic coloring," "hydrogenated," "pasteurized," "organically grown," and thousands of others simply didn't exist.

To navigate for safety in the modern diversity of foodstuffs, one must become an expert in critical thinking. Otherwise, how can you tell "organic" from "original," "sugar" from "sweetener," "real" from "natural," and solve countless other tricky puzzles for the sake of your safety? You have to constantly remember that the food industry stopped being your friend ever since the time of the Industrial Revolution, at which time it developed an ever-growing arsenal of creative means to deceive its customers with a sweet smile at the consumer's own expense. As a result, the majority of us face enormous problems connected to everyday eating.

The overwhelming majority of people today experience serious health problems. For example, 133 million Americans—almost one out of every two adults—has at least one chronic illness.[2] Nearly 70% of Americans take prescription drugs,[3] and over 35% are obese.[4] Based on available statistics, the number of perfectly healthy people in the United States seems to be rather low. Yet, similar to all creatures on planet Earth, all humans have a birthright to be healthy. Could it be that we don't spend enough money on our health? On the contrary, according to the World Health Organization, the United States spends almost $3 trillion a year on health care. So, what is missing? Do we need to develop more medicine? Maybe we are too busy? Or do we have to be more knowledgeable? How can we solve this mysterious paradox?

---

[2] "Chronic Diseases: The Leading Causes of Death and Disability in the United States," Centers for Disease Control and Prevention, last modified May 9, 2014, http://www.cdc.gov/chronicdisease/overview/index.htm.

[3] CBS News, "Study Shows 70 Percent of Americans Take Prescription Drugs," http://www.cbsnews.com/news/study-shows-70-percent-of-americans-take-prescription-drugs/.

[4] Nancy Hellmich, "U.S. Obesity Rate Levels Off, But Still an Epidemic," *USA Today*, October 18, 2013, http://www.usatoday.com/story/news/nation/2013/10/17/obesity-rate-levels-off/2895759/.

While I am not a medical doctor and cannot give medical advice, I have a right to share with other people my thoughts, observations, and concerns. I have been continuously and consciously researching natural health for over twenty years, and I have noticed a lot of contradictions between the real facts about human health, and the misleading claims made by food, drug, and medical industries. Based on my observations and research, I believe that you can significantly improve your health by applying the principles of natural healing. Yet it is only possible if you develop the ability for critical thinking and start to think for yourself. Otherwise, you become dependent on others to decide for you. In a sense you choose to stay blind. You follow someone else's instructions and perform actions that do not make much sense to you. You submit to the authority of others. You give your power away to the food, drug, and medical industries as well as to all of those who have a temptation to capitalize on your ignorance.

One time, my daughter Valya needed a wisdom tooth to be extracted. I offered to accompany her to the dental clinic, and Valya asked my opinion on what type of anesthesia she should select. When I was in my twenties, I had all four of my wisdom teeth extracted with local anesthesia. I clearly remember that it was a quick and easy procedure, after which I went straight to work. Other members of my family also had completely painless experiences under local anesthesia. Naturally, I recommended Valya to go for local anesthesia. I assured her that it would be a quick, easy, and safe process, especially considering that the dentists at this clinic specialized in tooth extractions. I advised my daughter not to worry at all.

On the day of her appointment, Valya arrived at the dental clinic relaxed and fearless; she joyfully told me about her art projects. After we filled out all the paperwork, the nurse invited us to a separate room, which was very white and cold. The nurse and Valya had the following conversation:

"So, you are going to do general anesthesia now?"

"No," Valya firmly replied, "I want local."

"You are so brave!" The nurse looked surprised.

"Why?" Valya asked.

"Because it could be very uncomfortable and painful!"

My daughter looked worried. The nurse continued, "You could possibly suffer from pain for several days; you will need to take strong painkillers."

"Please don't talk her into general anesthesia; she has already made her decision," I said.

"I just wanted the girl to know that it could be *very painful*." The nurse said firmly. "It is a complex procedure. Trust me, you don't want to be awake for this."

Then she left us alone in that cold room for about thirty minutes, and I noticed that my daughter was becoming nervous. I hugged her and reminded her, "Valya, you won't feel anything. I had my teeth extracted, and it was not painful at all."

Suddenly, the door opened, and in the hospital corridor the nurse was pushing a wheelchair with a teenage girl sleeping in it. The girl's face was very pale, and there was blood on her lips and chin. My daughter asked the nurse with a trembling voice, "Is that how I will look after my tooth extraction?"

"No," the nurse replied, "she had general anesthesia."

It was unfortunate for Valya to see that other patient right before her own surgery, and right at that particular moment our nurse told my daughter to follow her. I saw my daughter's wide-open, scared eyes, but I didn't have any time to give her my support. I went back to the waiting area. As I was waiting, more young people arrived for their wisdom teeth extractions. All of them chose to be "put under," as recommended.

Valya returned from surgery with a smile. She told me that the doctors were excellent, and the operation was quick and easy, and that during the entire surgery she felt no pain at all. Not even a pinch. We drove home from that clinic, glad that it was all over. Valya didn't have to take any medication after the numbness was gone on neither that day nor the following days. In about a week her gums healed without any complications. The only pain she felt came from the memories of fear and pressure she felt from the nurse. Valya was saddened at how many young people were manipulated with the use of fear into a more expensive, uncomfortable, and possibly more dangerous surgery.

In this story, many young people didn't have any way of knowing which anesthesia would be less uncomfortable, and, therefore, they chose what was recommended by professionals. However, I often receive emails similar to the following: "I have been consuming green smoothies for six months, and I feel great. But yesterday I read on the internet that green smoothies could be harmful in some way. Now I don't know what to do. Please help!" I feel helpless and have a hard time responding to these letters because I realize that no matter how objective and logical my answers are, they might be overridden in a matter of days by the next well-written counter claim.

An inability to apply critical thinking can potentially cancel the results of the best medical practices. Not long ago, my friend Caroline called from Los Angeles and told me, in tears, that drinking green smoothies didn't help her at all. Caroline then described to me that three months prior to that she discovered a small lump in her breast. She had a hard time deciding which treatment to choose, as there is a countless variety of clinics in Southern California. As a result, Caroline made appointments with an acupuncturist, a chiropractor, an herbalist, and a naturopath. Throughout that time my friend continued visiting her medical doctor "just to make sure"; she received a short course of radiation and took several prescribed medications as well as all of the herbs and supplements prescribed by her naturopathic doctors. During the same period, Caroline fasted for one week on juices and thirty-six hours on water. One of her doctors was concerned that she was not getting enough protein, so, following his advice, Caroline started eating grass-fed beef and chicken, immediately after her water fast. And that's not all she did. At the same time, my friend hired a psychic for a personal reading and booked a session with a famous astrologist. After three months of such "intensive care," her lump didn't go away, but instead enlarged. Caroline worked hard and spent a fortune on her treatments, but the results were negative. She felt devastated and didn't believe she could be healed at all.

This story illustrates how even the best therapies can be harmful if not consciously applied. Without comprehending what she was doing and the precise purpose of each procedure, this young woman was destined to follow other people's decisions. Since she could not choose between doctors and treatments, and she was afraid to miss out on the most important one, she decided to do all of them.

The above examples demonstrate the lack of ability to think for oneself. The statistics confirms that many people don't have such skills. In a recent surveying over 400 employers across the United States, it was reported that 70 percent of high school graduates were deficient in critical thinking.[5] Considering that only 75 percent of American students graduate from high school, we can estimate that the percentage of the people deficient in critical thinking is much higher, possibly over 80%.[6] I agree with American author Bryant McGill that "most people do not actually know how to think for themselves, and unfortunately that prevents them from even knowing it."[7] At this point the vicious cycle starts because, if I don't know how to think for myself and I don't realize that, whose advice do I follow? Besides thinking for myself I know only two options: to follow some authority or to follow the majority.

While it might feel safe *to follow the majority,* American psychologist Solomon Asch, through his classic conformity experiments, showed that about 75% of participants went along with the group's opinion for fear of being ridiculed or thought "peculiar," even though they did not really believe their conforming answers. (See detailed information on these experiments at simplypsychology.org.)

---

[5] The Conference Board, Corporate Voices for Working Families, The Partnership for 21st Century Skills, and the Society for Human Resource Management, *Are They Really Ready to Work? Employers' Perspectives on the Basic Knowledge and Applied Skills of New Entrants to the 21st Century Workforce,* 2006, 11, http://www.p21.org/storage/documents/FINAL_REPORT_PDF09-29-06.pdf.

[6] Gloria Bonilla-Santiago, "No Excuses: We Need 100 Percent High School Graduation," *STEM Education* (*U.S. News* blog), March 18, 2013, http://www.usnews.com/news/blogs/stem-education/2012/05/31/no-excuses-we-need-100-percent-high-school-graduation.

[7] Bryant McGill quotes, Goodreads, http://www.goodreads.com/author/quotes/5824390.Bryant_McGill.

Along with Asch, the scientists who conducted these experiments concluded that following the majority inhibits judgment. I would like to add that from my own observation, blindly following the majority brings loneliness and emptiness. I believe that following your own dream can make you feel happy and fulfilled, and you often need to swim against the current to accomplish it. That is the price of true happiness, and that is another big reason we need critical thinking.

What about following authority? In this book we talk about health, so let us figure out who is your primary authority on your health. Try answering these simple questions:

- Who has always been with you from your first breath and never left you?
- Who will always stay with you until your last breath?
- Who knows all your thoughts, your family history, and all the rest of your life obstacles?
- Who knows what you eat, how you sleep, and the rest of your habits, good and bad?
- Who knows all your health details, all the particulars of your organism, and if you ever got sick, who helped you to get well?

The answer to these questions is you, and nobody else. It is you who would most likely make the most accurate decision concerning your own health. Please note that I am not asking you not to visit your doctor or refuse every treatment your doctor recommends. Rather, I encourage you to start trusting yourself more and learn about the two main processes needed for human health: nourishment and detoxification. Then you can choose the most appropriate doctor and treatments according to your best adviser and authority—you.

When you trust your own judgment, you can learn a lot about your health. For example, it is safer to fast for a week and to see for yourself how you feel than to follow someone's recommendations without having any idea why you should. Through your own careful observations you have the ability to clearly see the results of your actions.

Critical thinking is a skill that has to be trained, preferably from childhood. Adults can develop their ability to think critically by observing, trusting what they see, and doing their own research. I insist that in most cases you can trust your own observations much more than those of any so-called authority. However, critical thinking trainers recommend that people develop critical thinking in a group, and there are also books, boot camps, and online courses available for those who are interested. A seven-day green smoothie cleanse in the company of your friends or relatives would be a wonderful opportunity to practice critical thinking. Throughout this book, I will try to invoke engagement in your own thinking. I hope to inspire you to observe which of your actions make you feel and look the healthiest and as a result create the best personal plan that works for you.

TWO
YOUR BODY IS ABLE TO HEAL ITSELF

I am alive! I mustn't forget it tonight, tomorrow, or the day after that.
—RAY BRADBURY

I remember when for the first time in my life I grasped the sense of the phrase "your body is able to heal itself." I heard it before but couldn't figure out what it meant. For a long time I thought it was unfair that some people would become ill and suffer, especially children. My oldest son was five then, and he was ill too much and too often. On the day he had his tonsils removed, I sat helplessly at his bed. My little boy was looking at me with his grown-up eyes on his pale face. I felt so much sorrow for my son's suffering that at times I couldn't breathe. On the way home from the hospital, a friend lent me a book, but only for one day. "You *must* read it," she said. I read Paul Bragg's *The Miracle of Fasting* in one sitting, and suddenly the day became brighter, even though my little son was still in the hospital. I read this book exactly one day too late when it came to coping with my son's illness. Perhaps I needed to go through a certain amount of pain before I could comprehend the simple truth: The body is able to heal itself!

In desperation I started translating the book into Russian and copying it over with a ballpoint pen on five stacks of extra-thin paper. I spent all day and all night writing. It made me feel better. When I ran out of blue ink, I continued with green, then with red. I was done at daybreak. I wished I could have made thousands of copies, but there were no photocopy machines in sight at that time. I had only five copies of my precious message to distribute to this town in the Moscow suburbs as it awoke. I carried each copy to friends I knew who could use this wisdom. I thought that, though I was late to save my own son from that unnecessary surgery, maybe my friends wouldn't miss their chance. That was the last time my son was seriously ill as a child. We became vegetarians, bought a juicer, and for many years forgot about disease.

It seems unbelievable to me now, but after our health improved and continued so for many years and in the midst of political changes in Russia, I lost the essence of my first discovery of the natural healing concept. Fifteen years later, in 1994, four members of my family became very ill, forcing me to look for the solution again. I rediscovered the same precious message through new books and from another perspective. Since then I have dedicated my life to researching and sharing the ways of natural healing and its core principle: The human body is able to heal itself because it is *alive*. When a bridge, a tower, or any other man-made structure breaks, it can never restore itself. If your house or your car gets the tiniest scratch, it cannot repair itself. Yet your body can; and it does repair itself whenever it's necessary.

Let's take a close look at a very common injury that we all have experienced. Imagine you cut a finger with a knife. Ah!

- Instantly, the sharp pain prompts you to drop everything and bring your attention to the injury.

- The blood starts flowing from inside out, washing out any possible dirt and bacteria from your wound.

- In a few seconds blood platelets gather at the site to form a clot, kind of like a natural bandage that will stay on the cut for a few days, protect your wound from any dirt, and help keep the edges of your skin together.

- As soon as this blood clot forms, the blood vessels widen, allowing maximum blood flow to the site, which causes inflammation. The reddish color of your skin and slight puffiness around the cut is a sign that white blood cells have started cleaning the wound of bacteria and other foreign agents that might have gotten in with that sharp knife.

- The repairs continue. New layers of collagen are laid under the cut. New capillaries are formed to serve as the new skin tissue.

- Contraction occurs at the edges of the wound, thereby reducing the size of the wound.

- Surface skin cells migrate from one side of the cut to the other, covering the wound with cells to form the new skin.

In most cases, within a week or two, the cut heals so smoothly that you cannot immediately find the place of injury on your finger. The body does its job perfectly. It can also repair more serious injuries, including bone fractures.

The human organism comes equipped with all the tools it needs to fix fractures. Doctors only support the body by creating the best possible conditions for healing. After that, the doctors stand back and give the body time to do its job. Sometimes the body heals a bone so well that it's impossible to tell the bone was ever broken. Simple fractures usually take about six to eight weeks to heal. The four main steps to bone repair are conducted, amazingly, by the human body:

- The blood vessels that ruptured in a broken bone cause a blood-filled swelling called a hematoma at the site of the fracture.

- A cartilaginous callus forms in place of the hematoma and acts as a splint for the broken bone.

- A bony callus forms, replacing the cartilage with a callus made of spongy bone.

- The bony callus remodels in response to stress placed on it, forming a strong, permanent patch at the fracture site.

Your body naturally knows how to perform these and numerous other operations. The natural balance when all parts of the body work in unison is called homeostasis. Similar to every living organism on our planet, the human organism is programmed to repair itself on a cellular level according to its intricate blueprints. I want to emphasize that your body is programmed to repair itself. You can count on it!

However, if you are deficient in vital nutrients, it might be challenging for your organism to heal itself. For example, to heal any bone disease the body needs magnesium, calcium, phosphorus, vitamins C, D, and K, and other nutrients. If it lacks these main components, then even the world's best doctors won't be able to help you heal without prescribing the missing nutrients first. Another major problem is a high level of toxicity in the environment and inside the human body. Toxins interfere with the normal functions of organs and make the process of healing hard or even impossible.

Therefore, I believe that there are only two main underlying causes for all illnesses in the world, *toxicity* and *deficiency*. In medical encyclopedias you can find descriptions of thousands of illnesses and conditions; however, the majority begin with deficiency and toxicity. If your body is poisoned with toxins and deficient in necessary nutrients, it simply cannot maintain homeostasis.

THREE

LIVING IN THIS TOXIC WORLD

Men become accustomed to poison by degrees

—VICTOR HUGO

When I explain in my lectures that we accumulate toxins in our bodies, often people look at me in disbelief: What toxins? Most people don't realize that we collect many pounds of toxic matter very quickly. Think, for example, about salt. When you add a pinch of it to your soup, it seems to be a negligible amount, especially when it dissolves in your meal and seems to disappear. However, think about how many packages of salt you buy in a year, and it sums up to at least several pounds. In addition, if you consume sugar, your total yearly intake could be measured in hundreds of pounds based on Americans' average consumption of 152 pounds of sugar in one year.[8] Even if you don't buy that much sugar, remember that it is found in countless foods, such as cakes, cookies, candy, and other sweets, as well as in ketchup, crackers, bread, soups, cereals, peanut butter, cured meats, salad dressings, and many others.

---

[8] "How Much Sugar Do You Eat? You May Be Surprised!" NH DHHS-DPHS-Health Promotion in Motion, July 2007, http://www.dhhs.state.nh.us/dphs/nhp/adults/documents/sugar.pdf.

Salt and sugar are only two examples out of 1,521 food additives as defined by the Codex Alimentarius Commission.[9] I invite you to stop for a moment now and try to imagine the mountain of chemicals and unhealthy substances that your own vulnerable body has to process in the course of your life.

I, too, for many years didn't realize how many toxins my body must process until one day I bought my own water distiller and cleaned one gallon of tap water in it. What I poured into the distiller looked like a perfectly clear liquid, officially considered good quality city water that most of my friends don't hesitate to drink. I expected to see a very small amount of white crystals left after the process of distilling (evaporating) this water. Instead, when I opened the distiller, I cried out and almost dropped it. There were all kinds of residue on the bottom, about two tablespoons of a dark brown liquid, about a teaspoon of gray gooey substance, and lots of white crystals on the sides. All of it smelled so intensely chemical that I was disgusted to touch it with my fingers and used gloves to wash the container.

I couldn't force myself to take showers in this water anymore and immediately ordered a water filter for my home, which I thoroughly researched.

I still cannot fully comprehend how all of these substances can be completely invisible in drinking water. Since this first experience, I have experimented with and distilled many different kinds of water sold in stores, and have understood for the first time in my life how polluted our water really is. Mind you, we have discussed salt, sugar, and water, only three possible sources of toxins out of thousands of others that poison our bodies. It is not my goal to frighten any of my readers. Rather, I think it is critical for everyone to try to comprehend how enormously toxic our modern world really is.

What can we do to minimize the damage to our organism from all of these toxins? Think how fast you can fill the wastebasket in your home.

---

9 The Codex Alimentarius Commission, established by FAO and WHO in 1963, develops harmonized international food standards, guidelines, and codes of practice to protect the health of consumers and ensure fair practices in the food trade, http://www.codexalimentarius.org.

Depending on the amount of waste, it could take a week, a day, and sometimes you may fill it within an hour. Similarly, by paying attention to the quality of your food and water, you unload your body from extra work and therefore greatly improve your health.

Because I underestimated the harm from synthetic additives, I used to think it time-consuming and annoying to look at the nutritional content on the back of boxes. At some point, though, I realized the devastating effect on human health, and that was when I started to consciously examine the ingredient lists on packaged foods with a small magnifying glass I began carrying in my purse. Soon I was able to evaluate any product or package with merely a quick glance, and I can now explain it to you in a simplified way. Let's take bread as an example because many people buy bread on a regular basis. I divide all breads into two main categories, the real ones and the fake ones. If you have ever baked at home, you know that the basic bread recipe contains only three or four ingredients: flour, water, and salt, or flour, water, culture, and salt. Such bread comes in dense, heavy loaves; it smells good and is nutritious. People have been consuming similar breads for many centuries without ill effects. The only minor problem is that this bread's shelf life is short at approximately two to three days.

The recipe that you see below is dramatically different. My friend who works for a bakery provided me with this recipe, and I promised not to disclose that bakery's name. I can only tell you that this bread is very popular and can be purchased at most supermarkets.

Whole wheat flour, water, high fructose corn syrup, wheat gluten, yeast, soybean oil, salt, calcium sulfate, extracts of malted barley and corn, honey, corn syrup, soy flour, dough conditioners (sodium stearoyl lactylate, calcium dioxide, ethoxylated mono and diglycerides, dicalcium phosphate, mono and diglycerides, datem and/or azodicarbonamide), yeast nutrients (ammonium phosphate, ammonium chloride, ammonium sulfate and/or monocalcium phosphate), enrichment (vitamin E acetate, ferrous sulfate, zinc oxide, calcium sulfate, niacin, vitamin D, pyridoxine hydrochloride, folic acid, thiamine mononitrate and vitamin B12), wheat starch, cornstarch, maltodextrin, vinegar, calcium propionate (to retain freshness), whey, soy lecithin.

Most of these ingredients are aimed at providing a longer shelf life (eight days), as well as making the loaf fluffier and seemingly bigger, while in reality it is quite light. While these qualities support the bread manufacturers' financial status, they contradict the nutritional purpose of this bread. A couple of slices of such bread would overload both your digestive and lymphatic systems for a few hours. Your organism will try its best to separate toxic substances from several grams of usable nutrients and send the toxins into elimination channels, such as those in the liver, kidneys, colon, skin, lungs, and others. Eliminating all of the toxic waste from these two slices of bread is a rather challenging task, and, if you start eating something else before the toxins from the bread are completely eliminated, the toxins from the bread will stay in your body indefinitely. And this could happen with each meal so that, if you consume foods that contain differing chemicals, the overall waste in your body will slowly but surely accumulate.

Toxicity (from the Greek *toxicon,* meaning poison) is the ability of natural and synthetic chemical compounds, in doses exceeding normal pharmacological levels, to induce the disruption of normal vital processes.[10] If we don't want to "induce disruption of normal vital processes" in our bodies, we should try consuming foods that are free from toxins. This is why I started looking at the ingredients lists on all cartons and packages of food I consider for purchase. Naturally, the assortment of packaged products that I allow myself to buy has shrunk to about a dozen. For my family I buy almost exclusively fresh or bulk products. If my friends or relatives ask me specifically to bring dessert from a health food store, I purchase some homemade local banana bread, nut bars, or something else that has minimal ingredients and zero preservatives in it. I have been following this course for many years and have even stopped noticing all other packages in the stores.

I consider myself to be a tough person; I have travelled and seen a lot of outrageous things in my life, from crocodiles in Africa to gigantic

---

[10] George Kvesitadze, Gia Khatisashvili, Tinatin Sadunishvili, Jeremy J. Ramsden, *Biochemical Mechanisms of Detoxification in Higher Plants: Basis of Phytoremediation* (Berlin, Germany: Springer, 2006), 2.

horseflies in Siberia. Still, I feel pain every time I watch a child eating some sugary dessert with some fifty toxic ingredients in it. For example, recently some close friends visited me, all three of them suffering with terrible illnesses. They are very kind individuals, and we enjoy talking for hours together. After we shared a nice healthy lunch, my friends brought a sack from their car, which was full of waffles and cookies of the worst kind. It was astonishing for me to watch them enjoying all of those toxic treats and immediately after our "healthy eating" discussions. Sadly, I see many people who seek and appreciate the information about nutritious foods but don't apply their knowledge to their real life. I observe this phenomenon again and again, as if talking is one thing and life is totally another. I would like to emphasize that if I say that processed foods are full of toxins, I really mean it. Even if it is perfectly legal to sell processed foods in supermarkets, these products are often dangerous to human health.

All sources of pollution are divided into two types: natural and anthropogenic, and technogenic, which result from human activities. "More than 500 million tons of chemicals are produced annually in the world. Wastes often serve as a source for the development of toxic microflora, which can transform them further into hazardous contaminants."[11] Food enhancers, trans fats, coloring, preservatives, pesticides, and other chemicals get into our bodies, and we absorb these and other toxic substances not only from our food but also from countless other sources. For example, each time you wash your dishes, especially if you use a dishwasher, some residue is left on them. The residue accumulates with each washing. Your food picks up part of the residue, especially if your meal is hot and you ingest it. What's more, dishwashing liquids are labeled "harmful if swallowed." Most contain diethanolamine, a liver poison, chlorophenylphenol, a toxic metabolic stimulant, or other dangerous toxins. At home I use only baking soda, hydrogen peroxide, or biodegradable soap for washing dishes.

I travel a lot and often stay in hotels. Once, I entered my room while the housekeeper was finishing up cleaning the kitchenette. I was

---

[11] Ibid, 1.

shocked to discover how she was cleaning the dishes. She washed them with a soapy sponge and placed them on a rack to air-dry without any rinsing. She explained to me that it was the standard procedure at this hotel and that the glasses would be shiny and easy to clean. Since then, every time I stay in a hotel, the first thing I do is wash all the glasses in my room with clean running water.

Another time, a man volunteered to help me in the kitchen at the retreat and began doing the same thing this hotel housekeeper was doing—washing our retreat glasses with soap and then leaving them to dry. When I insisted on rinsing the glasses, he tried explaining to me that all the soap would evaporate and the glasses would be a lot cleaner that way. I would like to debunk this myth once and for all. The clear chemicals are usually a hundred times more dangerous than what we call "dirt" itself. The food residue, especially when it is organic, is not deadly or poisonous, even though it looks messy. In fact, many cultures throughout history have used soil and clay to wash their bodies and clothes.[12] When you organize your retreat, try supplying natural cleaning supplies or biodegradable soaps for the sake of better detoxing and healing.

Another popular example of hidden poisons is the wide use of hand sanitizers. You see them everywhere, and, surprisingly, many people are using them. I have never used hand sanitizer even once and was not surprised to read on the CNN website the following:

> The main concern with hand sanitizers is triclosan, which is the main antibacterial ingredient in nonalcoholic hand sanitizers. "There's no good evidence that triclosan-containing products have a benefit," says Allison Aiello, associate professor of epidemiology at the University of Michigan. In Europe and the United States, hospitals won't even use them, she notes; it's thought that they don't reduce infections or illness. . . . Research has shown that triclosan

---

[12] History of soap, http://www.cleaninginstitute.org/clean_living/soaps__detergent_history.aspx.

can disrupt the endocrine system, amplifying testosterone. In animal studies, it reduced muscle strength. It may also harm the immune system.[13]

Little by little, countless noxious chemicals have penetrated all segments of our lives. If I attempted to write just one paragraph for each poison found in our households, it would result in a separate, multivolume book. Instead I urge you to pay attention to all possible sources of toxic poisoning in your life, such as preservatives in your nutritional supplements, cosmetics, shaving cream, shampoo, deodorant, particles of detergent in your clothes and linens, aspartame in your chewing gum, as well as the fumes from cars on the streets and at parking garages and so on. We live in a toxic world, but if we stay alert and apply our critical thinking, we can minimize our exposure to toxins almost to zero.

---

[13] Bob Barnett, "Is Hand Sanitizer Toxic?" *CNN Health*, October 16, 2013, http://www.cnn.com/2013/10/16/health/hand-sanitizer-toxic-upwave/.

FOUR

THE BEST SOURCE OF NOURISHMENT

The simple things are also the most extraordinary things,
and only the wise can see them.
— PAULO COELHO, *THE ALCHEMIST*

Green leaves conceal some of the greatest mysteries of nature that we have only begun to uncover little by little. Every spring trillions of beautiful green leaves come out of the soil and cover trees, bushes, and the ground. When I was a little girl, I wondered if people were able to cut as many leaves out of green paper with scissors. We are blessed that there is an abundance of leafy greens on our planet, and it doesn't cost us anything. All these precious greens are magically crafted out of sunlight, water, and soil to our eyes' delight and most importantly for our health.

Scientists still don't know all of the intricate nutrients that are contained in leafy greens, but what we already know is purely amazing. Apparently, greens are the most nutritious source of food on Earth, and that is why all creatures on our planet consume some form of greens. Even polar bears eat moss, tigers and lions munch on grass, and whales consume algae. Greens have been an essential part of the human diet since the beginning of time, but during the last two centuries people in Western countries have almost completely stopped eating them. There are still large groups of people in Africa, India, and other parts of the world, who rely on greens for their nutritional value. For example, according to the scientific research, "consumption of greens serves as a major source of vitamins and micro-nutrients for people that inhabit remote rural settlements near the Himalayas in India, where vegetable cultivation is not practiced and market supplies are not organized. Consumption of traditional diets known to these vegetarian societies is said to have many beneficial effects, such as prevention of age related degenerative diseases—arteriosclerosis, stroke, etc. According to several residents of this reserve, wild green leafy vegetables increase the amount of blood in the body which is likely to refer to the high iron content of many wild greens."[14] Furthermore, scientists from Norway conducted a chemical analysis of the nutrient composition of these greens and concluded that "green leaves were rich in energy, protein and minerals (calcium, iron) . . . in particular, rich in beta-carotene (3290 micrograms/100 g) . . . and that these traditional and locally produced green foods are valuable and important nutrient contributors in the diet both in rural and urban areas."[15] Finally, modern science confirms that greens can protect us against the worst human diseases.

CARDIOVASCULAR DISEASE

The consumption of green leafy vegetables has been demonstrated to reduce the risks associated with cardiovascular and other diseases.[16]

---

[14] Shalini Misra, R.K. Maikhuri, et al, "Wild Leafy Vegetables: A Study of Their Subsistence Dietetic Support to the Inhabitants of Nanda Devi Biosphere Reserve, India," *Journal of Ethnobiology and Ethnomedicine* 4 (2008): 15.

[15] M.B. Nordeide, A. Hatloy, M. Folling, E. Lied, A. Oshaug, "Nutrient composition and nutritional importance of green leaves and wild food resources in an agricultural district, Koutiala, in southern Mali," *International Journal of Food Sciences and Nutrition* 47, no. 6 (1996): 455–68, http://www.ncbi.nlm.nih.gov/pubmed/8933199?dopt=Abstract&holding= f1000,f1000m,isrctn.

[16] Melissa Johnson, et al, "Diets Containing Traditional and Novel Green Leafy Vegetables Improve Liver Fatty Acid Profiles of Spontaneously Hypertensive Rats," *Lipids in Health and Disease* 12 (2013): 168.

VARIOUS CANCERS

In the article "Foods that Fight Cancer," published by the American Institute for Cancer Research, scientists reported that "spinach, kale, romaine lettuce, leaf lettuce, mustard greens, collard greens, chicory and Swiss chard are excellent sources of fiber, folate and a wide range of carotenoids such as lutein and zeaxanthin, along with saponins and flavonoids. . . . Foods containing carotenoids protect against cancers. . . . The carotenoids in dark green leafy vegetables can inhibit the growth of certain types of breast cancer cells, skin cancer cells, lung cancer and stomach cancer. . . . Foods containing folate decrease risk of pancreatic cancer and . . . foods containing dietary fiber probably reduce one's chances of developing colorectal cancer."[17]

FOLATE DEFICIENCY

Another study discovered folates are available in a wide range of leafy green vegetables, while folate deficiency is a prevalent phenomenon worldwide.[18]

OXIDATIVE STRESS

"Varieties of cabbage and greens from the brassica family contribute as sources of important antioxidants and anti-inflammatory related to the prevention of chronic diseases associated to oxidative stress, such as in cancer and coronary artery disease."[19]

---

[17] "Foods That Fight Cancer: Dark Green Leafy Vegetables," *American Institute for Cancer Research*, http://preventcancer.aicr.org/site/PageServer?pagename=foodsthatfightcancer_leafy_vegetables.

[18] C. Wang, K.M. Riedl, and S.J. Schwartz, "A Liquid Chromatography-Tandem Mass Spectrometric Method for Quantitative Determination of Native 5-methyltetrahydrofolate and Its Polyglutamyl Derivatives in Raw Vegetables," *Journal of Chromatography B Analytical Technologies in the Biomedical and Life Sciences* 878, no. 29 (2010): 2949–58, http://www.ncbi.nlm.nih.gov/pubmed/20888309.

[19] S. Rokkaya, C.J. et al, "Cabbage (Brassica oleracea L. var. capitata) Phytochemicals with Antioxidant and Anti-inflammatory Potential," *Asian Pacific Journal of Cancer Prevention* 14, no. 11 (2013): 6657–62, http://www.ncbi.nlm.nih.gov/pubmed/24377584.

MACULAR DEGENERATION

Age-related macular degeneration (AMD) affects more than 1.75 million individuals in the United States. Macular degeneration is the leading cause of irreversible blindness among adults. American ophthalmology researchers conducted a study involving almost a thousand people and concluded that "those in the highest quintile of carotenoid intake had a 43% lower risk for AMD compared with those in the lowest quintile. Among the specific carotenoids, lutein and zeaxanthin, which are primarily obtained from dark green, leafy vegetables, were most strongly associated with a reduced risk for age-related macular degeneration."[20]

These studies represent only a tiny portion of some of the latest scientific research about the healing benefits of green leafy vegetables. I would like to share with you two of the most recent discoveries about greens that simply blew my mind.

MAGNESIUM

Over the last decade, several scientific studies have resulted in the discovery of the significant role of magnesium in human health. When I read the list of symptoms of magnesium deficiency, I was jumping and screaming because I have already noticed how many of these symptoms usually disappear as soon as people start consuming green smoothies on a regular basis. These recent discoveries have only confirmed what I have seen but didn't know how to explain. Now I am thrilled to share this information with you!

Green leaves are green because they are packed full of chlorophyll. Magnesium composes 6.7% of each molecule of chlorophyll and is located at the heart of this pigment-containing molecule. Without

---

[20] J.M. Seddon et al, "Dietary Carotenoids, Vitamins A, C, and E, and Advanced Age-Related Macular Degeneration. Eye Disease Case-Control Study Group," *Journal of the American Medical Association* 272, no. 18 (1994): 1413, http://www.ncbi.nlm.nih.gov/pubmed/7933422.

magnesium, chlorophyll would not be able to trap sunlight and harness its energy for plant growth during the process of photosynthesis.

New research published in the journal *BMC Bioinformatics* indicates that magnesium's role in human health and disease is far more significant and complicated than previously imagined. While it is well-known that all living things require magnesium, and that it is found in over three hundred enzymes in the human body, this new study indicates that a deficiency in magnesium may profoundly affect a far wider range of biological structures than previously understood. Listed below are seven key therapeutic applications for magnesium.

- Fibromyalgia: Not only is magnesium deficiency common in those diagnosed with fibromyalgia, but relatively low doses of magnesium have been clinically demonstrated to improve pain and tenderness in those to which it was administered.

- Atrial fibrillation: A number of studies now show that magnesium supplementation reduces atrial fibrillation.

- Type 2 diabetes: Magnesium deficiency is common in type 2 diabetics.

- Premenstrual syndrome: Magnesium deficiency has been observed in women affected by premenstrual syndrome.

- Cardiovascular disease and mortality: Low-serum magnesium concentrations predict cardiovascular and all-cause mortality.

- Migraine disorders: Blood magnesium levels have been found to be significantly lower in those who suffer from migraine attacks.

- Premature aging: Magnesium reduces the calcium that accumulates in soft tissues due to aging.

Please note the above mention of diabetes. You will read about the "miraculous" recoveries of diabetics in many of the letters at the end of this book.

VITAMIN K

This nutrient can be found almost exclusively in green leafy vegetables. All green leaves are abundant in this important, overlooked vitamin. Vitamin K deficiency has been linked to the following disorders:

skin cancer

liver cancer

heavy menstrual bleeding

nose bleeds

hemorrhaging

easy bruising

osteoporosis

hematomas

Vitamin K deficiency has also been linked to the following birth defects:

shortened fingers

cupped ears

flat nasal bridges

underdevelopment of the nose, mouth, and mid-face

mental retardation

neural tube defects

VITAMIN K2

Many people are not aware of the health benefits of vitamin K2. A study recently published by the European Prospective Investigation into Cancer and Nutrition (EPIC) has revealed that increased intake of vitamin K2 may reduce the risk of prostate cancer by 35%. Besides helping to prevent cancer, vitamin K2 is found to

- protect against heart disease;
- ensure healthy skin;
- form strong teeth and bones;
- promote brain function; and
- support growth and development.

While there is almost no vitamin K2 in greens or fruit, research in Canada demonstrated that consumption of Vitamin K positively influenced the formation of Vitamin K2 by human intestinal bacterium.[21] In other words, there is a possibility that regular consumption of green leafy vegetables may influence the intestinal flora in your body to produce vitamin K2.

These are only a few examples of the superiority of the nutritional content in green smoothies. I predict that many more amazing nutrients in green vegetables will be discovered in the future. Green smoothies are the easiest and most palatable way to consume large quantities of greens. The greens used in green smoothies belong to the most nutritious foods on the planet. During the seven-day green smoothie cleanse, you won't consume anything but green smoothies, which will allow your body to absorb a higher volume of nutrients, in contrast to regular eating, even when you add a quart of green smoothies daily.

---

[21] J.M. Conly et al, "The Contribution of Vitamin K2 (menaquinones) Produced by the Intestinal Microflora to Human Nutritional Requirements for Vitamin K," *American Journal of Gastroenterology* 89, no. 6 (1994): 915.

FIVE

DETOXING IS HEALING

The part can never be well unless the whole is well.
—PLATO

What would happen if someone accidentally swallowed some poison? That person would feel sick and would either vomit or develop diarrhea. Most people have had food poisoning or another similar experience in their lives at least once. Why do people feel sick after ingesting the poison? Obviously their organism is trying to remove the toxic substance from the body as quickly as possible. This function of the body is called the "detoxification process" or for short, "detox."

In order to better explain how detox works, let me draw an analogy. The process of accumulating toxins is similar to accumulating debt. Imagine some person, we'll call him Alex, borrowed $100. In one week, he paid back $30, but on the next day he borrowed another $50. His debt grew to $120. Alex worked hard, paid $40, but got a traffic ticket and had to borrow $75 more. His debt then became $155. After several years of such poor money-managing Alex found himself deeply in debt, working two jobs, tired, and unable to pay his debt off because his monthly wages were less than the interest on his debt. Luckily, Alex was able to declare bankruptcy so he could start to rebuild his credit.

The process of accumulating toxins in the human body is similar. Recall a time when you ate a not-so-healthy meal that contained some preservatives, gluten, white sugar, salt, and a little bit of pesticides. Your body needed about twelve hours to digest the edible parts and eliminate all the waste. Instead, you ate again six hours later. This new meal needed to be digested, so your body had to stop eliminating the by-products of the previous meal. Your body then needed more than twelve hours to completely clean itself of any waste products from both meals. Yet in two hours you had a coffee break, then in two more hours you partook in a dinner with friends, and another hour later you munched on popcorn at the movie theater. At that point, your organism required some serious time off from eating so it could finish the process of elimination of all the toxins from all these foods. You might have felt bloated, sleepy, or even experienced a headache. How many people realistically would know to stop eating once in a while for twenty to thirty hours? Instead, when feeling sluggish, most people reach for a cup of coffee, or a pill, and within a couple of hours they eat their lunch, then another one, and so on until one day the organism becomes ready for "bankruptcy"; in other words, the person "gets sick."

In nature, there is no constant availability of food for any creature. Only humans in the Western world have an opportunity to eat whatever and whenever they want. As a result, everyone's bodies are continuously accumulating excess particles from meals, but the majority of people don't realize they need to detox. Contrary to our human ignorance, the human body is very aware of the need to remove toxins from the body and attempts to perform a cleanse each time there is an opportunity to do so. For example, such a cleanse happens every night while we are sleeping.

This is not to say that detox starts only when you completely abstain from eating, such as when performing a water or juice fast. Getting rid of toxic waste is so imperative for your organism that it can start detoxing after a wide range of events in your life, such as adding workouts to your routine, improving your diet, or vacationing for a few days. In order to detox, your organism not only needs extra energy but also some inner "workforce," which includes several conditions, such as a blood flow that is free from urgent tasks and is available to carry oxygen, hormones, and nutrients. The lymphatic system should not be overloaded with toxins. The liver, kidneys, and other elimination organs must be in good shape and able to take on a load of cleaning work. The digestive tract must have healthy bacteria, function with good peristalsis, and be free of constipation. Even though these factors are obviously necessary for an effective detox process, unfortunately, these conditions are extremely rare because most people have never been taught about the importance of regular detoxing. So our organisms have been forced to detox a little from time to time whenever possible. Every time a little extra energy becomes available, the organism applies it toward detoxing. That is why we often become ill during the first couple of days of our vacations, including children.

I invite you to educate yourself and experiment and observe how your beautiful body uses every opportunity to remove toxins. In order to start experiencing detox symptoms, you need to improve your lifestyle to a healthier level in any possible way. I have seen people developing detox symptoms from just removing white sugar from their diet, from switching to an organic shampoo, from having an enema or colonic irrigation, from installing a water filter in their kitchen, from starting to wear natural organic fibers, or even from beginning to sleep on a firmer mattress. Please don't just believe me, but instead try to see for yourself.

Detox symptoms may include any of the known symptoms of the so-called diseases. Some of them include white coating on the tongue, bloating, irritability, skin rash, headache, trouble sleeping, nightmares, diarrhea, constipation, drowsiness, low energy, congestion, mucus discharge, and fever. All these detox signs may seem awful, but in the vast majority of cases the symptoms are pretty mild. They usually don't last longer than a day or two, and, after the unpleasant sensations are over, people feel more youthful and energetic. I hope you wake up in the morning and say, "Wow! I haven't been feeling so good for such a long time that I didn't even know I could feel this good now." From my observations, healing without any unpleasant symptoms at all is not possible because they are caused by your body's efforts to expel toxins. All you can do to help eliminate those toxins faster is by resting, fasting, and managing stress. You can read more about the detox process in some of the letters at the end of this book.

If anybody in the world can heal you, it is your own body. It is wonderful that you don't have to pay your body to heal you. You don't need to have insurance to cover your body's work for you. It is fully committed to your well-being. The ability of the body to detox itself is a blessing that has saved countless lives. I greatly appreciate this gift and hope that you do too. It is very important to learn to appreciate the detox process and even to celebrate its manifestation. At our retreats we teach participants that if someone expresses symptoms of headache or congestion to reply with a smile and say, "Congratulations, your body is detoxing!" Indeed, we should be grateful for the amazing ability of our organisms to self-cleanse.

Our bodies are dedicated to our survival, not our death. The disease-like conditions that our bodies create, such as coughing, sneezing, fever, pain of different kinds, or high blood pressure, are nothing but the body's effort to survive. Ironically, when the body heals after taking pills, it most likely heals not because of but in spite of the medicine. I feel sad that such a great misunderstanding exists even among many health professionals. I wish science would do more research on how to help the body heal itself instead of treating the symptoms. By suppressing symptoms, we counteract the wise efforts of the intelligent human body. Our organisms are always ready to act on our behalf, and they never make mistakes. If we listen carefully to our bodies, we can all know what we need to do to feel better.

SIX

MANAGING STRESS

Your body hears everything your mind says.
—NAOMI JUDD

Earlier in this book I said that there are only two main underlying causes for all illnesses in the world, toxicity and deficiency. However, for those who don't know how to manage it, stress can become the third cause of disease. Countless stress management techniques exist in the world, and they work for many people. I particularly like The Work of Byron Katie, a system that teaches to "love what is." In the past, we have incorporated this program in several of our green smoothie retreats and have been discussing the importance of finding one's mission in life. You can learn more about The Work program at www.theWork.com.

People inevitably develop stress if they do not follow their dreams. Among hundreds of participants, I never met anyone who didn't have a dream, but very few people follow it in their real life. I have observed that, without following your personal dream, your life can become empty, meaningless, and even depressing. Many people try replacing emptiness with pleasure or fun, but it never works because no matter how much fun one has every night, or during the weekends, the feeling of wasting one's life remains. At a young age, most people think that their dream is not important, or it can wait until they become established in life, so they go to work, which they often don't care for, and after work they go somewhere "to have fun," or "to rest." The words "TGI Friday" reflect this desperate attempt to recover from a week of empty labor. That neglect of one's dream is the main reason for everyone's stress.

On the other hand, I have met people who do follow their dreams. I have noticed that even if they are tired, hungry, poor, or even in physical pain, they still look content, and their smile is emanating from their entire being. You have a birthright to do what you desire, to think what you enjoy thinking about, and to be with people you enjoy being with. That is the true wealth of this world, and stress management doesn't substitute for it.

At our retreats we talk about our true desires, and many participants discover that they have never taken the time to find out what they really want in life. All of us have been influenced and manipulated by the media and advertisements into thinking that we want money, wealth, fame, and other similar things that seem so obviously attractive that it never occurred to us to question all those fake dreams, which, on their own, don't make anyone truly happy. For some of our participants it takes several hours to write one sentence on a piece of paper about what they really dream about. Many people have confided with me that they had never thought about it before. It seems that for them a weeklong retreat is a perfect place for deep and long conversations with friends.

I may surprise you by stating that the physical health that you gain during a healing retreat is not the most important part of the experience. The significance of a successful retreat involves the profound insights that you gain during the event. Have you ever had an "aha" moment? This occurs when you have a sudden insight or realization of great life significance. Furthermore, an aha moment is a comprehension that allows you to look at life or a situation in a completely different way. A good retreat is always full of aha moments in which hundreds of questions arise in your head while observing the process of your own detoxing and healing. I think these new insights have even more value than the physical rejuvenation people get at healing retreats.

How else can you reduce stress, especially if you suddenly became disappointed with something? I recommend any form of exercise; you will feel good as soon as you start your workout. Your body will begin raising the level of endorphins—one of the "feel good" chemicals in the brain—and you will feel calm and balanced. I prefer walking because the rhythmic promenade in nature always brings profound thoughts to my mind. Also, walking is the most natural movement for all humans, and it is good both for the body and the mind.

SEVEN

EDUCATIONAL MATERIALS FOR YOUR RETREAT

Education is the kindling of a flame, not the filling of a vessel.
—SOCRATES

At our retreats, we teach several classes daily in which we discuss theory about natural healing and encourage people to find examples from their personal experience. When you perform your own seven-day green smoothie retreat, we encourage you to read books and watch videotapes that will correlate with your personal experiences and observations. The combination of learning from books and your personal aha moments is the best foundation for your comprehension and application of natural healing. Then you will never be afraid of your bodily functions. You won't panic when you suddenly experience pain or other distress. You will be able to choose your own strategy for how you can best support your body to heal from any condition.

As you contemplate organizing your own green smoothie retreat, I highly recommend that you watch the following three videos:

- "The Seven Best Green Smoothies" by Valya Boutenko. Following the procedures in this video will ensure the highest quality and deliciousness of your green smoothies.

- "The Miracle of Greens" by Sergei Boutenko. This video will inspire you and get you excited about your green smoothie retreat.
- "Reversing the Irreversible" by Valya Boutenko. This documentary will inspire you to improve your health via natural means.

I also recommend that you browse our YouTube channel, which is called "Boutenko Films." On this channel, you will find several hundred short videos, many of which are testimonials from participants of our green smoothie retreats.

Attitude is very important in every endeavor. Promoting inspiration during a green smoothie retreat provides participants with support and helps to complete the task, especially if they experience challenges with the program. Engage yourself in activities that provide you with support and keep you inspired, such as:

- watch other people's testimonials about green smoothies online;
- read books about green smoothies on your own;
- read a chapter once or twice a day aloud and discuss it in your group;
- before each meal read aloud to your group nutritional facts from the Internet or from Valya's phone app called "Quality Produce"— you will be amazed at the healing properties of fruits and greens;
- rent or download and watch together educational videos, and discuss them afterward; and
- talk to people who regularly drink green smoothies.

Having a small library of books about green smoothies and natural healing on hand will also help you during your green smoothie retreat. Reading these books will help you to better understand the process of detoxing and healing. By the end of the cleanse you will be able to relate to most of the information in these books and can start writing your own. For ideas on which books to read please check out the bibliography at the end of this book. At the same time, however, you don't want to overload yourself with information. Sometimes, you may enjoy watching a nice, heart-warming comedy. Rent or download several comedies ahead of time. Laughter is another great healer for you.

Reading and watching documentaries is important, but you will be learning as much if not more from observing each other's healing progress. For example, consider what Diane McCann from South Australia wrote about her retreat:

> I attended the green smoothie retreat in Australia and I felt absolutely fantastic at the end of the week. More energy, more life force and a clearer head, but what amazed me more were the people who were very unwell to begin with. For example, I was shocked to observe the lady with bad arthritis, whose fingers unfurled at the end of seven days. My roommate's need for insulin reduced dramatically in seven days and her eyes went from yellow inside the lower lids to healthy pink. Everyone at our retreat had miraculous shifts in health, energy, and positivity. I have been drinking green smoothies daily ever since and that was three years ago.

EIGHT

WHY GREEN SMOOTHIES?

A green smoothie a day keeps the doctor away.
—SERGEI BOUTENKO

In my family, we like to fast 24–36 hours each week on water, juices, or green smoothies. Of the different types of fasting that we have tried, the green smoothie cleanse is our favorite due to its outstanding results. A green smoothie retreat is the optimal format to detox and be nourished because green smoothies are cleansing and super nutritious at the same time.

We eat to gain energy. Paradoxically, the very process of digesting food utilizes up to 30% of your body's energy.[22] Maybe you noticed that you feel sleepy after some heavy meals. On the other hand, when you eat lightly or have a break between meals for several hours, your body saves energy and often applies it toward inner cleansing. For the same reason, many people have an unpleasant taste in their mouth upon awakening in the morning, along with stiffness, headache, puffy face, crusty eyes, and other signs of detoxing at night.

---

[22] Helen Kollias, "Research Review: A Calorie Isn't a Calorie," Precision Nutrition, http://www.precisionnutrition.com/digesting-whole-vs-processed-foods.

The more toxic our food is, the bigger effort it takes to remove this poisonous waste from our organisms. After all eliminative channels become full of waste, some toxins get pushed into the spaces deep within vital organs, such as brain tissue, nerve cells, capillaries, bone marrow, and other places. The detoxing process usually starts after you haven't eaten for several hours. The body begins to remove toxic matter from tissues all over the organism into the eliminating channels, such as lungs, skin, liver, kidneys, and the digestive tract. The longer you abstain from eating, the more thorough your detoxing is. Therefore, to perform a detox on a deeper level, the body needs more time than one night of sleep.

The high fiber content of green smoothies makes you feel full for several hours after each smoothie. Without fiber, complete elimination is nearly impossible, The human body is built miraculously in such a way that almost all the toxins from every part of the body, including millions of dead cells, daily end up in the human sewage system—the colon. The colon fills up with waste matter so full of poison that we look at it with disgust, not daring to touch it. In order to eliminate this matter, the body needs fiber. If we do not consume fiber, most of the toxic waste accumulates in our body, and most of the toxins are directed to the bowels. We have to eliminate many pounds of toxins regularly.

The lymphatic system performs detoxing on a much deeper level than the colon does. We can call the lymph fluid "the river of life" as it keeps flowing in your body all your life, protecting it from pathogens and toxins. According to Dr. Samuel West, if the lymph ever stops flowing, the body dies in less than 24 hours. The cleaner your lymphatic system is, the stronger your immunity. The lymphatic system drains fluid from various parts of the body and carries microscopic waste through the lymph nodes, where the lymph is cleared from pathogens and toxins. The cleared lymph is emptied back into the bloodstream and circulates around the body once more.

During your seven-day green smoothie cleanse, you will go through a deep detoxing process on many levels. As soon as your lymphatic system, liver, kidneys, and other organs participating in digestion are freed from most of the toxic waste, the absorption of important nutrients increases manifold, causing the nourishment that is necessary to repair your inner organs. You will then start to feel and look younger. Often, our participants tell us that their relatives, who come to the airports to pick them up after the retreat, are shocked with the participants' youthful appearance. After one woman's seven-day green smoothie retreat in Australia, her own mother passed her by because she looked ten years younger!

Another factor that makes a green smoothie retreat optimal for your nourishment includes the beneficial consumption of green smoothies four to five times daily. Green smoothies are digested quickly, usually in less than an hour. The body quickly removes an excess of water-soluble nutrients, such as most of the vitamin B family and vitamin C, and any intake above the usable amount will be excreted with the urine. At the same time, vitamin C and other acid-based nutrients are antioxidants that perform important tasks, such as neutralizing free radicals, lowering blood pressure, and fighting off viruses and infection. By consuming green smoothies four to five times a day for seven days straight, we reintroduce these important nutrients again and again into our system (I recommend sipping green smoothies slowly rather than gulping them quickly).

Contrary to many other kinds of fasting, the longer you live on green smoothies, the easier it becomes. I know many people who initially wanted to try going on green smoothies for a few days and instead they lived on green smoothies for many weeks or months. A friend of mine named Clent M. lived on green smoothies for one year and reversed all of his major health problems. Most people say that only the first couple of days are challenging. If you manage to keep on a program through the first few days, it becomes much easier and pleasant.

NINE

FRUIT: TO EAT OR NOT TO EAT?

One must ask children and birds how cherries and strawberries taste.
—JOHANN WOLFGANG VON GOETHE

To eat or not to eat fruit—this is one of the most confusing topics in today's natural health field. Several raw food leaders recommend almost completely eliminating fruit from one's diet. At the same time, other experts suggest eating twenty bananas a day. Who is correct? In my opinion both sides have valid truth to their views.

Recently I visited several big cities in the Midwest of the United States: Chicago, Detroit, Cleveland, and others. While looking for ingredients for my own green smoothies I visited many different stores. I was deeply distressed to witness the poor variety and condition of produce in general, and fruits in particular. Some stores had some organic produce, but many of them had none. The farmers' markets also had little to zero organic produce. I was able to find greens that were not wilted, but I could hardly find any ripe, organic fruit—no wonder my smoothies were so tasteless as only my strong belief in their goodness made it possible for me to drink them.

The apples, peaches, and pears were all unripe, hard as a rock, and had no aroma or flavor. The berries and grapes were not ripe, and most were moldy. The oranges and kiwis were unripe and sour. I asked several people to describe the taste of an orange; they all said it was sour. Every time I visited a store in the Midwest my heart went out to all of the customers. I thought, how can I suggest people make green smoothies if the majority of people don't have access to healthy produce?

Unfortunately, on the other hand, I have discovered that there has been little scientific study done on the nutritional benefits of tree-ripened fruit. There are, however, many articles written by vegetarians, raw foodists, and other people for whom fruits serve an important part of their diets. For example, Valentina Borisenko, from the Siberian city of Irkutsk in Russia, spends half the year in Indonesia because she feels a lot healthier "at the place where she can consume plenty of tree-ripened fruit."[23] I believe that the fruit's vine is not unlike a vessel transmitting mother's breast milk to a child. We all know that the longer a baby is nursed by the mother, the healthier the baby is. Similarly, if the fruit is allowed to ripen on the mother-vine, basking in the sun, this fruit undoubtedly will contain superior nutrition.

To illustrate this effect, I will share a personal story with you. Prior to my arrival in Thailand, Valya, who arrived a day earlier, prepared sliced fruit for me, knowing that I would be hungry after a sixteen-hour flight. Valya was asleep when I came in at 3:00 a.m., but I found a plate of fruit next to my bed. I tried the fruit, and it was so scrumptious that I was sure I had never tried it before. I was curious and in the morning asked Valya what it was. She looked at me with her big round eyes, shrugged her shoulders, and said, "Those were mangos and bananas." It appears that the taste of the same fruit when it's ripe as opposed to unripe is vastly different.

Having been a raw foodist for twenty years, I have learned that I don't thrive on unripe, conventionally grown fruit. As such, every summer I go to "U-pick" farms in order to get tree or vine-ripened fruit,

---

[23] "Why Is It So Important to Eat Ripe Fruit?" Fruitarian.ru (blog), http://fruitarian.ru/pochemu-tak-vazhno-est-spelye-frukty.

both temperate and tropical, and I have noticed several obvious traits of vine-ripened fruit.

- It has a strong, pleasant smell.
- The skin is thin and easy to peel off.
- The taste is distinctive and rich.
- Most humans find the taste of ripe fruit enjoyable.
- Fruit flies and insects fly around the fruit.
- The seeds are dark.
- When I consume ripe fruit, I feel satisfied for several hours.

Some of you might say that it is impossible to distribute vine-ripened fruit in stores. I used to believe that too. This year I visited twenty-one countries, and of course I shopped for produce everywhere. I discovered that in some countries fruit was expensive and scarce; however, the quality was much higher than in most of the supermarkets in the American Midwest. Even in Eastern European and Northern European countries I was able to find superb-quality raspberries, wild strawberries, and ripe *seeded* grapes. Apricots were so ripe they were almost clear, and they were juicy and sweet. I was especially amazed at the deliciousness of plums; I had become so used to their plain, sour taste when conventionally grown that I had stopped buying them in my hometown.

I also interviewed several diabetics in Europe who described how their blood sugar was not affected by the consumption of ripe, organic fruit. On the other hand, if they consumed unripe, conventionally grown fruit, they had to inject more insulin. That surprised me because I always thought the riper the fruit, the more sugar it would contain. The only explanation I can think of is that in ripe, organic fruit, the sugar comes with important co-factors that enable the body to absorb the sugars with less negative side effects, so I completely understand how eating only unripe, conventionally grown fruit might be considered harmful to your health. Therefore, I propose that scientists do more research on the nutritional comparison between ripe and unripe fruit.

If you live in a warm region, you are blessed with the ready availability of ripe fruit. For those who live in colder climates, getting ripe fruit is more challenging. Some of you might wonder, what can I do if I don't have access to high-quality fruit? First of all, become aware. Second, go to U-pick farms in the summer and freeze berries and fruit for your winter consumption. Third, talk to your local farmers, and see if they can help you find a way to access organic produce. Finally, consider growing your own fruit.

It is my opinion that fruit, if it's ripe and organic, is an essential part of the human diet. Furthermore, I believe that no human can receive adequate nutrition without the consumption of high-quality fruit. However, I don't recommend a completely fruitarian diet because it is not complete. Again, greens are the most nutritious food on our planet. In my food pyramid greens take first place—so I try to get as many wild greens as possible—and ripe organic fruit takes second.

TEN
WILD EDIBLES

What is a weed? A plant whose virtues have never been discovered.
—RALPH WALDO EMERSON

Wild edibles in most instances contain more vitamins and minerals than commercially marketed plants do. Weeds have not been "spoiled" by farmers' care in contrast to the cultivated plants in the garden. In order to survive in spite of constant weeding, digging out, and spraying, weeds have had to develop strong survival properties. For example, in order to stay alive without being watered, most weeds have developed unbelievably long roots. If you have ever tried to pull a dandelion plant with the roots, you understand what I mean. Alfalfa roots grow up to twenty feet long, reaching for the most fertile layers of the soil. As a result, all wild plants, whose weeds have not been disturbed, possess more nutrients than commercially grown plants. I was so silly when I always used to pull out the "nasty" lambs-quarters from my garden to let my "precious" iceberg lettuce grow.

However, a word of caution is in order. Because of some poisonous plants in nature, we must be careful when picking wild edibles. While there are countless benefits associated with eating wild foods, there are also some risks, and I urge you to *take caution when harvesting wild foods.* It is a good idea to first learn how to positively identify edible plants. Visit the library or your local bookstore, and find a book that pertains to your local area. Eating wild edibles is fun, healthful, and safe when done properly, but please take the time to educate yourself and your loved ones. If you are ever in doubt about whether a plant is edible or not, don't eat it!

The best way to learn which weeds are edible is to sign up for an herb walk with an experienced guide in your local area. This way you can learn to recognize particular edible plants by actually touching, smelling, and tasting them so that you can gather your "wild produce" on your own. Also, there are lots of articles and photos of edible weeds on the Internet. You can also read Sergei Boutenko's book *Wild Edibles* to learn about how wild edibles are the only authentic food available on our planet.

Some of the most nutritious plants have thorns on their stems and leaves. I understand that, if they didn't have such protection, they would be extinct by now because animals would favor these plants for their nutrition. I have often successfully added stinging nettles and cactuses to my green smoothies. It is interesting that such thorny plants contain very little or no alkaloids, which makes them a valuable addition to our diet. Of course, we need to use some kind of gloves to handle them. After they are blended they don't sting at all.

To find out from reliable sources if there really is any significant nutritional value in dandelions and other weeds, I calculated all the numbers using the latest and most trustworthy scientific data. I was astounded at the results of my research. Compare the numbers yourself in the following two tables.

In the left-hand table I have listed the essential minerals and vitamins found in 100 grams of green leaf lettuce. On the right I have listed the essential minerals and vitamins found in 100 grams of dandelion greens. Note how much more nutritious the dandelion greens are in comparison to green leaf lettuce. For example, as seen from the third-column (the percent daily value), just 100 grams of dandelion greens more than meets your daily need of vitamin A at 203%. It also supplies 58% of your daily need of vitamin C, 19 % of calcium, a whopping 973% of vitamin K as well as a whole lot of other essential nutrients.

LETTUCE, GREEN LEAF, RAW	**DANDELION GREENS, RAW**
Serving size: 100g	Serving size: 100g
Amounts Per	Amounts Per

Vitamins Selected Serving %DV

Vitamin A 7404IU 148%	Vitamin A 10,160IU 203%
Vitamin C 18.0mg 30%	Vitamin C 35.0mg 58%
Vitamin D ~ ~	Vitamin D ~ ~
Vitamin E* 0.3mg 1%	Vitamin E* 3.4mg 17%
Vitamin K 174=mcg 217%	Vitamin K 778mcg 973%
Thiamin 0.1mg 5%	Thiamin 0.2mg 13%
Riboflavin 0.1mg 5%	Riboflavin 0.3mg 15%
Niacin 0.4mg 2%	Niacin 0.8mg 4%
Vitamin B6 0.1mg 4%	Vitamin B6 0.3mg 13%
Folate 38.0mcg 10%	Folate 27.0mcg 7%
Vitamin B12 0.0mcg 0%	Vitamin B12 0.0mcg 0%
Pantothenic Acid 0.1mg 1%	Pantothenic Acid 0.1mg 1%
Choline 13.4mg	Choline 35.3mg
Betaine 0.2mg	Betaine ~
Amounts Per	Amounts Per

Minerals Selected Serving %DV

Calcium 36.0mg 4%	Calcium 187mg 19%
Iron 0.9mg 5%	Iron 3.1mg 17%
Magnesium 13.0mg 3%	Magnesium 36.0mg 9%
Phosphorus 29.0mg 3%	Phosphorus 66.0mg 7%
Potassium 194mg 6%	Potassium 397mg 11%
Sodium 28.0mg 1%	Sodium 76.0mg 3%
Zinc 0.2mg 1%	Zinc 0.4mg 3%
Copper 0.0mg 1%	Copper 0.2mg 9%
Manganese 0.3mg 13%	Manganese 0.3mg 17%
Selenium 0.6mcg 1%	Selenium 0.5mcg 1%
Fluoride ~	Fluoride ~

* Alpha tocopherol

Do you still want to pull the dandelions out of your garden? By adding wild edibles to your meals, you can further increase the variety of greens in your diet and rotate them constantly for better nutritional results.

ELEVEN

CHOOSING THE BEST TIME FOR YOUR RETREAT

The future starts today, not tomorrow.
—POPE JOHN PAUL II

When is the best time for you to do a healing cleanse? When asked this question, Paul Bragg always replied, "The best day is today!" I agree that it's wise to do your cleanse sooner rather than later. However, it might take at least a couple of weeks for you to prepare well in order to get the best results. First, read this book, prepare the necessary equipment and ingredients, find companions, arrange a venue, and then you are ready to go.

How often should you conduct a green smoothie retreat? After you succeed in your first retreat, I recommend you conduct one every three months, particularly in the beginning of spring and fall seasons to prepare your organism for seasonal changes. If you live in a cold climate area, I recommend that you conduct your retreat during the warm season, so that you can benefit from the best-quality produce at reasonable prices.

Sometimes people share with me that they don't want to "sacrifice" their long-awaited vacations for a healing retreat. Such fears come mostly from those who have never participated in a healing retreat.

Once you have had the enjoyable experience of a green smoothie retreat, you will always look forward to another opportunity to become healthier, younger, and happier. Traditionally, vacationers go to resorts located near beaches in warm climatic zones where they spend several days lying in the sun in long chairs, covered with toxic sun screen, eating lots of fast food, and drinking alcohol and soft drinks. Such vacations are costly but make almost no difference in the vacationer's health and often make people more tired and depressed.

I also go to the resorts from time to time. Only, I organize my vacation time according to my own standards. I always carry with me a small "travelling" blender, along with a paring knife and a couple of small bowls wrapped in a kitchen towel. Whether it is Fiji, Thailand, or Mexico, on the day of arrival, I hire a taxi to go to the local farmers' market and buy lots of ripe fruits and greens. From that time on, my vacation begins to roll in the direction of health and joy.

Sometimes people ask if they could live entirely on green smoothies. While I think it is beneficial to conduct weeklong green smoothie retreats as often as you wish, I don't recommend going on a green smoothie diet lasting many months and years. First of all, the ingredients in green smoothies do not cover all the nutrients that we need for our own individual nourishment. The list of such nutrients is particular to each of us and is also different from region to region. You also don't want to adapt your digestive tract to exclusively liquid food. Finally, you need to eat carrots, apples, nuts, and some other solid foods that you need to chew, as sufficient chewing is important for many functions of your body. So, the primary goal in your eating plan should be to maintain a balance between health-giving green smoothies and the rest of your diet.

TWELVE

CREATING A RESTFUL ENVIRONMENT

What is without periods of rest will not endure.

—OVID

For our retreats we always choose resorts that are located away from big cities, with plenty of fresh air. Often these grounds have limited access to the Internet and cell phones, which is a benefit for our guests. We absolutely exclude any television or radio, which we substitute with viewing a carefully selected list of DVDs and audiotapes. We also make sure that the only food available within a walking distance is our own, and we pay special attention to the quality of beds and bedrooms to ensure all participants' quality rest at night.

Most people have experienced in their lives both good and bad night's sleep and know the difference one feels in the morning. After a night of disturbed sleep, in which you cannot fall asleep for a long time, wake up many times during the night, or experience nightmares, you may wake up tired and miserable. If you have had too few hours of sleep, you may feel desperate for more sleep and angry at your alarm clock. However, when you have had a good night of sound sleep, you wake up peaceful, contented, and energized. You feel like a happy child, strong and smiley. That is how important a good night's rest is.

There are many causes of sleepless nights. For example, the consumption of coffee alone contributes to shallow, disrupted sleep.[24] After a stressful day, people retire with a bundle of disturbing thoughts in their minds. Lack of exercise, heavy foods, especially before bed, problems in personal relationships, and nutritional deficiencies can also contribute to inadequate rest.

Nighttime is when the body prefers to heal and detox. In fact, that is the only time the body has to perform most of its own healing. Have you noticed that when you go to bed with a toothache, headache, itching, swelling, or other discomfort in your body, you tend to wake up in the morning with less pain or sometimes completely without distress? That is a result of the natural healing process that happens at night. Unfortunately, very few people in the world enjoy a good restful sleep. For example, 30% of American workers don't get enough sleep.[25] In addition to a lack of sleep, most people also experience poor quality of sleep in general.

Lack of sleep accumulates and interferes with the body's natural ability to restore itself. While we cannot often change the circumstances of our everyday lives, we can compensate for some of the lack of sleep during the seven-day green smoothie retreat. Not only can you sleep as many hours as you desire, but your body also rests from the energy-consuming task of digestion. With each day of your cleanse, your body becomes more and more free from toxins, which allows your organs to regenerate. When your organs are healed, they work more efficiently. The overall better condition of your inner organs greatly contributes to your feeling of vitality.

However, despite drinking wonderful green smoothies, during the seven-day cleanse people often complain that they don't sleep at night. This happens when the body is loaded with toxins, and the process of detox intensifies. Even if you don't want to sleep, try to stay in bed lying

---

[24] Caffeine Dependence (website), http://www.caffeinedependence.org.

[25] Sara E. Luckhaupt, "Short Sleep Duration among Workers—United States, 2010," *Morbidity and Mortality Weekly Report* (Centers for Disease Control and Prevention) 61, no. 16 (April 27, 2012): 281–285, http://www.cdc.gov/mmwr/preview/mmwrhtml/mm6116a2.htm.

down with your eyes closed. Usually it happens for only one or two nights; after that, people sleep noticeably better. The following recommendations will help you sleep better.

- Whenever possible, sleep in the fresh air; fresh outside air is rich in negative ions. Elevated negative air ion levels are widely reported to have beneficial effects on humans including enhanced feelings of relaxation and reduced levels of tiredness, stress, irritability, depression, and tension.

- Let your energy field restore. Our energy field expands several feet beyond our body in the shape of a gigantic egg. This energy field is our cradle of healing. At night any damage is repaired, but not if we have alarm clocks next to our heads or computers running in our bedrooms. All electrical devices and electronic gadgets have an electromagnetic field that also extends out for several feet beyond their physical structures. When the two fields cross, the body cannot fully heal. I personally turn off all electrical fixtures and move electronic gadgets to another room. I'm also careful about refrigerators, microwaves, or other strong devices running in an adjacent room because the plywood wall does not stop those harmful vibrations.

- Sleep on a hard surface; our bodies need to stretch out at night. Our bones and joints can only stretch out when we lie on hard surfaces. This is especially important for the spine. During the day, the spine is improperly positioned while driving, sitting in front of the computer, and watching TV, and some spinal joints don't get adequate spinal fluid and blood enriched with oxygen. My entire family prefers to sleep on hard beds or on the floor in sleeping bags. If we are forced to sleep on soft beds, we wake up with headaches and feel achy and unrested.

Over the years, I have received many comments from our participants that after the seven-day green smoothie retreat they felt rested for many months, and their sleep was sounder.

THIRTEEN

WHY SEVEN DAYS?

Oh, the difference between nearly right and exactly right.
—H. JACKSON BROWN, JR.

In August 2013 my family and I conducted the nineteenth green smoothie retreat. This time it was in Canada. Before green smoothie retreats, we conducted approximately forty other different kinds of retreats, such as raw food retreats, juice-fasting retreats, water-fasting retreats, and spiritual retreats. Some were weekend retreats, or two-, three-, four-, and five-day retreats. I began to notice that two, three, four, and even five days were not enough, mainly because of the detoxing process. When we were doing four- or five-day retreats, many of our participants were leaving at the peak of their detoxing process, with headaches, fevers, nausea, and other discomforts. Obviously, that was discouraging. During seven-day retreats, on the other hand, most people complete the first cycle of detoxification and feel significant improvement. They all experienced discoveries and some profound aha moments. In addition to their own healing, people witnessed thirty or forty other participants reversing some conditions with which they have been suffering for a long time.

You might ask if it makes sense to do retreats longer than seven days. However, I don't recommend that because your daily smoothies eventually begin to feel routine, boring, and never-ending. Sometimes people choose to go longer than a week, for example, in cases where someone's detox has not finished and they enjoy the process and feel comfortable continuing for longer. In such cases, people individually go for two, three, or four weeks on green smoothies. My friend Clent M. decided to live on green smoothies for an entire year after his doctor told him that he had only two weeks to live. You can read his story in my book *Green Smoothie Revolution*.

Seven days is the natural measure of time; the moon cycle is twenty-eight days, and one week is exactly a quarter of the moon cycle. This fact has found its place in most traditional religions and philosophies in the world. The rest of this chapter focuses on, from my personal reflections, how each of the days of the weeklong green smoothie retreat progresses for most participants.

On the first day, everyone is excited and scared at the same time. They are still connected to their work, families, and world events through their phone calls and thoughts, emails, etc. It is usually disturbing and somewhat frightening for people to leave the habitual rhythm of life and yield to the new, slower healing mode. For this reason, we usually make an effort to surround our newcomers with maximum attention, delicious green smoothies, and uplifting lectures and organize positive entertainment, such as live music or motivating documentaries.

On the second day, many participants are surprised to wake up with headaches and stuffy noses. Usually people become disappointed, and some even panic. To comfort our participants, we explain in our presentations the importance of the detox process and encourage them to appreciate and embrace detox symptoms. By the end of the second day, roughly two-thirds of the people develop one or another sign of cleansing.

The third day can be the hardest day of the week for most people. It is understandable because they feel hungry, sick, and often slightly depressed and tired. That day, we usually go from person to person and listen to them while trying to engage in warm dialogue and reassure them that all the discomfort is a good and normal sign. This is an opportunity for people to carefully observe their personal process of healing and every part of their transformation to understand how the body restores its homeostasis. It is very important for them not to get distracted from this learning experience, but to consciously observe all the activity that happens within their organism. On that day, we encourage people to share with each other how they feel in detail and to write about it in their journals.

The fourth day can still be hard for many people; however, there are always a few who have already passed the peak of their detox. They show up to the green smoothie breakfast with a big smile and announce, "I feel like a million bucks!" or "I don't remember ever feeling as well as I do now!" Or they state, "The numbness in my left foot that I had for ten years is gone!" Or, "My cravings for smoking have disappeared!" Or, "I never slept so well in my life!" And so on. On that day, we intensify our exercise program and provide more information in all our classes.

The fifth day is when most people feel profound improvement. They still have minor symptoms of detox, but they notice that their health has positively improved and they like their reflection in the mirror. Everybody experiences the presence of extra energy, clearer thinking, improved vision, and the ability to concentrate. This is the best day for learning. We encourage people to read more, attend all the lectures, and exercise actively as well as engage in dialogue with all the other participants in order to exchange unique and valuable information.

On the sixth day, most people feel even better. Many people comment that they haven't felt this great since their teens. They begin to ask many questions; they want to learn more about this cleanse in order to share with others. They feel happy and inspired.

The seventh day is a day of total happiness and love. Most people sense groundbreaking accomplishment on that day. Everyone feels like a hero: "I made it! I believe that my body can heal me!" People are grateful for the amazing experience. They usually comment that their hunger is completely gone, and they begin to drink fewer smoothies and feel more satisfied. These observations are extremely important as many people come to green smoothie retreats fearing they'll suffer from not being able to eat habitual food. Contrary to that expectation, by the end of the week most participants feel accustomed to healthy eating. The body becomes used to eating healthy and begins to crave healthy food. People say, "I can do it!" which is more than they initially anticipated from this retreat.

These types of results are why I recommend the seven-day green smoothie retreat. How could I possibly take away any of these days?

FOURTEEN

DAILY SCHEDULE

Whatever begun with planning, ends in a victory.
—AMIT KALANTRI

When you make the decision to conduct a green smoothie retreat, write a detailed plan at least a couple of days prior to beginning your program, because after the retreat starts it's not a good idea to leave your sanctuary, especially for minor things you may have overlooked.

You can start with creating a seven-day calendar. The below is a sample of one day's schedule.

6:00—Good morning!

6:15—Practice some morning yoga or other exercise.

7:00—Prepare the first green smoothie for breakfast.

7:30—Have breakfast.

8:15—Go for a walk.

9:00—Read a chapter from a book and discuss.

11:00—Walk or do some other exercise.

11:30—Prepare a green smoothie lunch.

12:00—Have lunch.

1:00—Enjoy some free time.

2:00—Watch a video about natural health and discuss.

3:30—Prepare a green smoothie dinner.

4:00—Have dinner.

5:00—Practice breathing exercises.

5:30—Enjoy some free time.

6:30—Prepare a green smoothie pudding for supper.

7:00—Have supper.

7:30—Watch a comedy.

9:00—Go for a walk.

9:30—Night-night!

You can adjust these recommendations to fit your needs.

Try including exercise or walking two to three times a day. I don't believe that you need to lie in bed to conserve energy. On the contrary, you need to activate your lymphatic system for better detoxing. Sometimes you will feel low energy and no desire to move at all. If you overcome that and start walking slowly, within a few short moments your lymph will start moving through your body and you will feel more energy and pleasant sensations in all your limbs. Of course, at times, there may be exceptions from this recommendation when you decide to stay in bed. You will understand what I am trying to describe if you start regularly exercising from the first days of your retreat.

You can add free time, meditation, daytime naps, singing, listening to music, or any other activities. I strongly urge against any TV-watching, however, because it could distract you from your healing, detoxing, and resting.

FIFTEEN

KEEPING A DIARY OR BLOG

Keep a diary, and someday it'll keep you.
—MAE WEST

I encourage you to keep a diary throughout your green smoothie retreat. (I prefer spiral-bound notebooks for my personal diary.) Your diary is your closest friend and companion with whom you can share your most intimate observations. Writing in a diary will also help you cope with your detox symptoms. For example, if you ever feel sick, you can read your diary and be inspired to heal naturally. Whenever you decide to conduct another green smoothie retreat for yourself, you can prepare yourself better by reading your diary. Also, if you ever decide to write a book or just an essay for a blog, your diary will be helpful in composing an inspiring story based on facts. Finally, you won't know how helpful and enjoyable a diary can be until you start one.

Along with keeping notes in your diary, you can also keep a log-book of your measurements. To measure yourself, you will need a tailor's measuring tape, a notebook, a pen, and a scale.

Copy the following list into your notebook.

circumference

upper arms, left and right

neck

bust

waist

hips

thighs, left and right

calves, left and right

weight

Measure the circumference of each of these parts of your body and write the result next to each item. The first time you measure yourself, it will take some time, but as you become familiar it will go more quickly. Measure yourself every day at the same time, or have someone else measure you. I recommend that you do it upon arising from bed for accuracy. Taking measurements will become an important and reliable support tool. Keeping all the support you possibly can will combat any challenging moments and temptations.

Also in your diary or blog, list your best-tasting recipes from your retreat. Start creating your own compilation of green smoothie recipes. Share and trade your recipes with other friends.

Similar to a diary, a blog can be inspiring and helpful during and after the retreat. While it is less intimate, a blog is open to potentially countless other people. Think about how many times in your life you have found inspiration from other people's blogs. Other advantages of a blog are that it cannot be physically lost and you can benefit from the comments from other people to instigate further exploration of your topics. What I like about my blog is that I write only a page or two once a week, but throughout the months I accumulate a great quantity of information that is helpful for reference, especially when someone asks me for my opinion.

With the abundance of smart gadgets today, you may enjoy starting a video blog or a podcast. You can videotape yourself talking about your cleanse daily, as well as interview your partners. It is a fun way of learning because "teaching is the highest form of understanding," according to Aristotle. Finally, a video blog will keep you occupied and add fun to your entire project.

SIXTEEN

THE IMPORTANCE OF SUPPORT

Alone we can do so little; together we can do so much.
—HELEN KELLER

Inviting a couple of other people to your retreat instead of doing it alone can provide you with psychological support as well as help with blending, cleaning, shopping, and other tasks.

One can always go on a seven-day cleanse alone, I have done it many times by myself, and many people do that. However, including other people in your program ensures the successful completion of your intended cleanse. Read below what Robert and Mary N. wrote about their experience at one of our retreats.

On the first couple of days most people felt symptoms of a detox. After only three to four days we all started feeling unbelievable. Similarly, the other people changed too and started to look healthier, more energetic, and more balanced. It was amazing to observe in others what we felt internally. All participants opened up and shared about their personal experiences, which were changing day-by-day. We felt confident that our health was continually improving with every glass of wonderful, healthy smoothie.

When you are on your own, you may quit on the second or third day after experiencing minor detox symptoms or after having some doubts or stressful thoughts. When you participate in a project as a group, it takes a serious problem for you to quit in the middle.

In my family, when one of us announces a desire to go on even a short-term, one- or two-day fast, somebody else in the family often joins that person just for support. In fact, recently I was doing my own personal green smoothie cleanse when family members, including my brother and my nephew who live in Canada, joined me for one or two days during different periods of my cleanse. That felt very nice because I had somebody to talk to about the particulars of my healing. With my family support I easily stayed on green smoothies for eighteen days. At the same time, I was happy to inspire my loved ones to benefit from short smoothie fasts.

I have noticed that whenever people go on a cleansing program, they love to discuss in detail all their bodily functions, new sensations in their organism, difficulties, concerns, and achievements. People who are not doing a cleanse get not only bored quickly but also irritated, possibly because they regret that they are missing the benefits of the cleanse. For that reason, at our retreats we discourage participants from calling home too often and sharing in detail their personal transformations, which are not always easy. Relatives of our participants have confided with me many times that they found some of the details disturbing, alarming, and even disgusting.

Doing a cleanse as a group makes the task of preparing smoothies many times easier. It's almost the same amount of work, whether you make a smoothie for one or for three people, because it involves practically the same amount of blending and cleaning. Also, you can take turns preparing fresh smoothies at different times of the day. I strongly recommend that you prepare a fresh smoothie four times a day. This is necessary to keep your taste buds and spirits entertained without getting bored.

In my family, we know that Valya makes the yummiest green puddings, Sergei is good at savory green soups, and I am best at super-green smoothies. Similarly, before working in the kitchen with a group of helpers at each retreat, we let everybody make various smoothies at different times and then decide together who is good at what. Since Sergei is a morning person and enjoys making the first smoothie of the day, he shows up at the kitchen at dawn, turns on pleasant music, and prepares his "bucket o'smoothie" while tapping his feet. Dagmar, my helper at Swedish retreats, prefers to be the last one in the kitchen, so she always helps with the last smoothie of the day. Some people prefer to take care of one smoothie all by themselves. Others like to work in pairs so they can talk. We always try to share the work in a way that leaves everybody most satisfied. Among our team that operates in the kitchen during the green smoothie retreats, some people prefer to chop the produce while others favor blending, and there is usually someone who wants to do the cleaning job in his or her own way.

If you want to be able to fully concentrate on your healing, and if your budget allows it, you can hire another person to do the blending and cleaning of the kitchen. Also, adding a couple people to your retreat will enable you to buy produce in bulk, and you will save not only on produce but also on gas. In addition, you can afford to buy a larger variety and better quality of produce, which further enhances your green smoothie experience.

SEVENTEEN

THE COST OF PRODUCE FOR YOUR RETREAT

Pay the farmer now, or pay the doctor later.
—ANONYMOUS

Shopping for ingredients for green smoothies must be discussed ahead of time. Ask your partners if they have any special sources for produce, such as gardeners in the neighborhood, friends, farmers, or special deals and discounts. Ask who has a bigger vehicle because the boxes of produce take up a lot of space. Optimally, greens and berries should be purchased every other day. Most of the fruit can be purchased for the entire week ahead of time. The below is an approximate list of foods that you may want to consider purchasing.

Greens

arugula	collard greens	dandelion greens
green leaf lettuce	kale	mitsuna
mustard greens	red leaf lettuce	romaine lettuce
spinach	Swiss chard	

Herbs

basil	cilantro	mint
parsley	sunflower sprouts	

Vegetables and fruits

apples	apricots	bananas
berries (wide variety)	cucumbers	kiwis
lemons	mangos	melons
oranges	papayas	peaches
pears	persimmons	pineapples
plums	tomatoes	watermelons

Seeds/miscellaneous

chia seeds	dates	dulse flakes
psyllium husk powder		

I encourage you to use the best possible quality of produce. We have discussed that deficiency is one of the two major underlying causes of disease. At a green smoothie retreat, you have the opportunity to focus on nourishing your body, and, as you are detoxing, your assimilation of nutrients increases. Even if you have to pay double price for better-quality produce, I believe it's worth it. I always go for the best quality, organically grown, and as wide a variety as possible, with a big preference for dandelion greens, sorrel, and other wild edibles. For the highest nutritional content, I select younger plants with smaller leaves. The best quality produce is your true health insurance.

WATER SUPPLY

In 2013 I visited several regions in the world where centenarians live in the highest density. Centenarians are people who are over a hundred years old. At each site we took samples of water, which we tested at a lab. The tests showed that centenarians consume water that is the lowest in calcium—under 12 milligrams per liter. As soon as I returned home to the United States, that is when I purchased a water distiller, and now I consume only distilled water because I too want to be a centenarian. If you are able to use distilled water, I recommend it highly. If not, use the purest water you can find. At our retreats we usually provide both pure water and lemon water, which is prepared by adding approximately one or two teaspoons of freshly squeezed lemon (or lime) juice to each quart of water. Lemons and limes contain unique flavonoid compounds that have antioxidant and anti-cancer properties. Lemon juice also makes lymphatic fluid thinner, which helps to remove toxins faster, and helps eliminate extra calcium from the body, making some detox symptoms milder.

I don't think it is possible to purchase all the produce necessary for the entire week as well as ensure its freshness for seven days. Usually, we have a delivery of fresh produce three to four times during our weeklong retreats. To calculate the quantities of produce you need for one week,

- measure first how much produce is used to prepare one quart (or liter) of green smoothie;
- multiply this amount by four to figure out how much you need per day per person;
- multiply by the number of participants; and
- multiply by seven to get the total amount of greens and fruit you need for the entire week for your group.

If your budget allows, then go to the best health food store you can find in your neighborhood and buy the highest-quality produce. If you have to watch your budget, however, there are several ways you can save money. While the produce in the store can be outstandingly expensive, you can always find free, or almost free, adequately good fruits and greens:

- Order in bulk at wholesale prices.
- Buy directly from local farmers.
- Go to U-pick fields and gardens.
- Learn to recognize and pick wild edibles.
- Talk to your neighbors who grow an abundance of fruit and cannot consume it all.

At most stores, you can order both fruits and greens by the case at a 10–30% discount, depending on store policy. If you're hesitant to buy large quantities of different ingredients, you can for sure buy a case of bananas and a case of apples for your one-week retreat.

When my son Sergei was a teenager, he grew sprouts and some produce for local health food stores. To determine a retail price, the stores added 30–40% to the cost they paid him. It is the same with local farmers: if you go directly to your local farms and buy in large quantities from them, you can ask for a 30–40% discount. The bonus of that will be that you will get the freshest-picked produce.

U-pick organic gardens are a fun outdoor activity. I enjoy going with family or a friend, and in one hour I gather a bucket of strawberries, a large basket of blueberries, or several buckets of pears of superb quality at a fraction of retail prices.

In my family, we almost never buy greens from early spring to fall when we have dandelions, lambs-quarters, chickweed, purslane, and stinging nettles in our backyard and in the local park. I love my wild edibles and prefer to have them in my smoothies over the store-bought greens that have been cultivated by humans over centuries. Cultivated greens have lost their bitterness along with some of their nutritional value. Again, if you would like to learn more about wild edibles, I recommend Sergei's book *Wild Edibles*. You can also purchase his Wild Edibles app on your iPhone or Android, and use it while foraging right in the park.

While it is uncommon these days to walk around and talk to neighbors, I encourage you to try it. I have lived in several locations in my life, and at every location, while taking hikes, I noticed many fruit trees in nearby yards. In the summer, I noticed ripe plums, figs, or pears fallen from the trees and bushes in abundance, just lying on the ground. When I talked to the homeowners, they greeted me with a smile and told me they were happy for me take some of these fruits. This is how I get scrumptious figs, perfectly ripe peaches, cherries, and pears that are beyond compare to what I can get in the store. And the price is right! In appreciation, I bring a jug of green smoothie, a bowl of fruit salad, or my new book to these neighbors, which makes them even happier.

I invite you to be creative when making arrangements for financing your program. For example, I did a one-week juice fast with my friend Peggy who paid for the cabin that we rented with her credit card because she had a special deal that then saved us almost half the cost. I gladly took care of the produce cost. Another time, a person who participated in our retreat had no money to pay us, but he offered to forage for fresh edible wild greens daily. Every morning this young man got up early and brought two buckets full of freshly picked weeds. Everyone in the group appreciated that.

When planning your produce purchases, don't forget to make arrangements for food deliveries. It is not advisable for you and your participants of a green smoothie retreat to leave the chosen sanctuary, whether it is a specially rented hotel, resort, or at home. You might encounter challenges and temptations that can be hard to overcome. In addition, you will have a very special psychological climate within your group, and reentering the world can completely erase the positive "vibes." You might start thinking about your work, politics, relationships, or placing phone calls, which makes it difficult to return to the healing mindset. To combat these challenges, you can ask your relatives or friends to help you with delivery, or arrange delivery from the store or farmer. Most stores even offer free delivery with a large purchase.

EIGHTEEN

EQUIPMENT FOR YOUR RETREAT

The equipment you've got really dictates what you're going to do.
—MARIANNE FAITHFULL

In addition to food, you will need some equipment for your green smoothie retreat.

a strong blender

large bowls for produce

knives

cutting boards

pitchers, glass jars with lids, and glasses for green smoothies

citrus juicer for preparing lemon water and juice for recipes

high counters

natural cleaning supplies

refrigerator space

compost bucket

flower vase (optional)

A strong blender

A high-speed blender is best, but if you don't have one of your own, try to borrow one from a friend.

Large bowls for produce

You will need four or five large bowls (2–3 gallons) or any containers for washing and cutting your fruits and greens before blending. I prefer to use stainless steal bowls, but at different retreats we have used glass or food-grade plastic containers. You can purchase them at restaurant equipment stores.

Knives

We usually use two to three small knives for paring and one medium or large knife for cutting greens and large fruit, such as melons and watermelons.

Cutting boards

Try using wooden cutting boards to avoid toxicity from plastic.

Pitchers, glass jars with lids,
and glasses for green smoothies

At green smoothie retreats we use almost exclusively glass for all dishes in which we pour smoothies. We use glass pitchers, glass jars with lids, and glass cups for serving smoothies. We never use disposable dishes, especially Styrofoam or plastic cups. It is a scientifically proven fact that plastic leaches into the food.[26] Usually during the week of the cleanse, many people become sensitive to smells and can taste the plastic in their green smoothies and water. Of course it takes more effort to clean glass, but at our retreats we choose to wash fifty glasses four times a day for the sake of health and ecology. We have found it best to use tall glasses, approximately 18 ounces, as this size seems to be the

---

[26] Jon Hamilton, "Study: Most Plastics Leach Hormone-Like Chemicals," *NPR.org*, March 2, 2011, http://www.npr.org/2011/03/02/134196209/study-most-plastics-leach-hormone-like-chemicals.

satisfying amount for everyone. At the first retreat, we served 8-ounce cups, and people had to run back and forth several times to fill them.

High counters

After facilitating many retreats we have learned the importance of having high counters. Preparing green smoothies involves lots of peeling, chopping, and slicing. You don't want to add backache from working in the kitchen to your detox symptoms.

Natural cleaning supplies

During the course of retreats, people often become super sensitive to strong smells. Also, we have already discussed that toxicity is another cause for disease. During the cleansing process, it is best to eliminate toxic substances from use in the kitchen. Therefore, at our retreats we use only natural cleaning supplies such as distilled vinegar, hydrogen peroxide, baking soda, and biodegradable soap.

Refrigerator space

At our retreats we use walk-in coolers because we usually go through twenty to thirty boxes of greens and fruit. For a retreat for 3–4 people, one standard household refrigerator should be enough. Keep only greens and overripe fruit in the fridge. Fruit that is not overripe doesn't need to be refrigerated. In fact, some of your fruit, such as pears or bananas, will only ripen at a warm temperature.

Compost bucket

Prepare for tons of compost. At our retreat we fill two 30-gallon garbage cans with compost daily. You might produce two or three buckets of compost per day on your retreat. If you try putting all your compost in the trash, your garbage will be extremely heavy, leaky, and smelly. Additionally, scraps from green smoothie retreats constitute high-quality compost, and it is a pity to send them to the landfill. At some resorts where we don't have a composting process, we make arrangements to drive our compost to the woods and bury it in the soil. With the current rate of soil erosion in the world, we feel obligated to return nutrition back to the earth. *Important:* It will save you a lot of effort if you arrange for your compost provisions while you are looking for the venue for your retreat. I encourage you to find places where you can dispose of your compost daily.

If you have some land, you can keep the compost for your own garden. Dig a trench about 12 inches deep (30 centimeters), throw in the compost items, chop and mix with soil, then cover with more soil. In a few months the rotted material will have been incorporated into the ground, and you can plant your vegetables into the now enriched soil. If you have a raised-bed garden, you can dump the food scraps into the raised bed and push them deep into the soil so that no scavengers can get to them. In no time the worms will have digested every last bit of the food scraps! An earthworm produces its weight in castings daily.[27]

Finally, we hope that you recycle cardboard boxes and other materials that come with your produce. I am proud to say that at our retreat in Sweden we have zero garbage as a result of a well-organized recycling process.

Flower vase (optional)

We love to surround ourselves with flowers at our retreats. If you don't like cut flowers, you can decorate your retreat with flowers in pots and planters. Usually we combine flowers into large bright bouquets and display them in the dining room and lecture hall. This creates a special-event atmosphere and uplifts everyone's spirits. You don't want to spend your retreat in a gray and monotonous environment. Flowers are the easiest technique to brighten your mood.

---

[27] "Earthworms," Kansas State University Research and Extension, http://www.hfrr.ksu.edu/doc1749.ashx.

VARIETY AND QUANTITY OF SMOOTHIES

Nothing is pleasant that is not spiced with variety.

—FRANCIS BACON

At our retreats we serve green smoothies four times a day. We make sweet green smoothies for breakfast at 8:00 a.m. and for dinner at 4:00 p.m. We serve savory green soup at noon for lunch, and we always finish the day with a green smoothie pudding at 7:00 p.m. As such, we do not limit consumption to three meals per day, but we provide only one 8-ounce cup of pudding in the evening, because we don't want people to overeat before bedtime.

On the first day of the green smoothie retreat, we purposely put extra fruit that is ripe in our smoothies to ensure that the smoothies are sweet, delicious, and enjoyable for everyone. These smoothies may contain 60–70% fruit. As the retreat progresses and everyone's blood sugar level begins to drop and participants become more sensitive to the sweet taste, we gradually reduce the amount of fruit in our smoothies. By the fourth and fifth day, the volume of greens in our smoothies reaches 50%, and on the sixth and seventh day they reach 70% and sometimes even 80%.

In most cases, a green smoothie should contain only three ingredients: greens, fruit, and water. The only exception is one we make for puddings in order to thicken the texture in pudding recipes—we add either psyllium husks or chia seeds. Another benefit of these two ingredients is that both psyllium husks and chia seeds help with elimination, which is important during this retreat.

We have noticed that everybody feels different about savory green soups. Some people adore them, and others cannot tolerate them at all. Also, some participants prefer spicy soups, while others choose very little spice or even blandness. To accommodate everyone we have created a special technique. We blend and pour in a separate pitcher a mixture that we call the "super spicy mixture." We place it on the table next to the bucket with the plain green soup, and everybody adds the spicy solution according to their liking. To make this super spicy mixture, we pour a couple cups of the regular smoothie into the blender and add lots of spices to it. The spicy smoothie can be created with garlic, hot peppers, gingerroot, mustard greens, turmeric, and so on. Sample recipes of spicy blends are provided in the recipe section along with some of our best green smoothie recipes. Please use our recipes as ideas that you can expand on and improve to your liking.

TWENTY

RE-ENTERING THE WORLD

You have brains in your head. You have feet in your shoes. You can steer yourself in any direction you choose.

—DR. SEUSS

On the seventh day of living on green smoothies most people feel exceptionally well, and, of course, they intend to continue staying healthy and, possibly, improving their health even further. The typical question that arises is, "How do we keep the achieved level of health? Do we have to stay on green smoothies for the rest of our lives?"

As long as you continue eating wholesome food, without any preservatives, flavorings, or other chemicals you will enjoy vibrant health. After over twenty years of research, I have developed a highly raw diet, which works well for my family as well as for the majority of people I know, and this way of eating is relatively easy to maintain. The below figure is my personal food pyramid.

I encourage you to always prepare your own meals from scratch and recommend having a large green smoothie for breakfast. I assure you that it is much easier than you can imagine, and, by the time you finish your weeklong green smoothie retreat, you will become an expert on blending green drinks. To get you started, I have supplied fifty basic

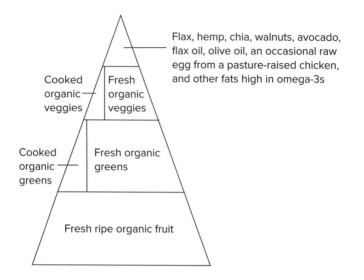

Flax, hemp, chia, walnuts, avocado, flax oil, olive oil, an occasional raw egg from a pasture-raised chicken, and other fats high in omega-3s

Cooked organic veggies

Fresh organic veggies

Cooked organic greens

Fresh organic greens

Fresh ripe organic fruit

green smoothie recipes in the recipe section of this book. A big green smoothie daily is going to be your most nutritious meal in your meal plan. And I hope you will keep this green habit for the rest of your life.

You can prepare a big salad for lunch from a wide variety of ingredients. Explore the assortment of veggies at all your local health food stores and farmers' markets. Make a goal of tasting every single piece of produce available, which will ensure that you are getting the most nutrients possible and enjoying tasty meals to the maximum. You can find some of my family's favorite salad recipes in the recipe section, but remember that these are just basic ideas that can be varied indefinitely.

For dinner I suggest a salad accompanied by some baked or steamed veggies, such as a slice of pumpkin or squash, yams, asparagus, beets, cabbage, cauliflower, string beans, celery, kale, bok choy, mushrooms, tomatoes, or other veggies. I usually squeeze a little lemon juice or a teaspoon of oil on my cooked veggies. Also, I often like to prepare a simple veggie soup for dinner, which is unbelievably easy and fast to prepare. It is a big mystery for me why chefs at so many restaurants keep adding flour to their soups, as well as other ingredients that are plainly unhealthy. There is absolutely no justified reason to add flour, oil, bouillon cubes, MSG, stabilizers, and other rather toxic items to our meals. In fact, soups taste far better without any of these added ingredients. Many of our friends who have tried our soups are greatly surprised by their outstanding deliciousness. Often people who otherwise habitually dine at restaurants claim that they could live on our soups for the rest of their lives. In the recipe section of this book you can find some of our simple and delicious soup recipes. Don't be alarmed by the seeming over-simplicity of some recipes. Just try making them, and I promise you won't be disappointed.

One of the most common and urgent questions I am asked is about animal food consumption, vitamin B12 deficiency, and other issues connected to the vegan and vegetarian diet. I was a strict vegan for ten years and not able to avoid a B12 deficiency. Since I started adding an occasional raw egg from pasture-raised chickens to my diet in 2008, my B12 levels have become normal. Some of you may be disappointed by this modification, and I completely appreciate your position. I only want to be honest and speak the truth about my personal experience.

The meal plan that I describe in this chapter has been working well for my family for several years now, and I would like, once again, to emphasize the major role of daily green smoothies in this plan. So, happy blending to you!

PART TWO

Letters from Our Retreat Participants

GREEN SMOOTHIE BABY

When I started my journey to health in August of 2010, my weight was 216 pounds. I was ill and depressed. I was diagnosed with polycystic ovary syndrome (PCOS), insulin resistance, anemia, and I had my period only once or twice a year. This was possibly the darkest part of my life. Thank goodness for a friend of mine who lent me a DVD on raw foods, which gave me light at the end of my very dark tunnel.

After I watched the documentary about the benefits of a raw foods diet, I googled "raw foods" and soon came across the book *Green Smoothie Revolution*. Since the day I bought my Vitamix blender I have had a green smoothie every day. Drinking all these green smoothies gave me boundless amounts of energy. I was walking up to 12 kilometers a day, and as I got lighter I started running that distance.

By Easter 2011 I was down to 143 pounds and attended the green smoothie retreat where I lost another 6 pounds in seven days. I was down to a US size 2 in clothes and had a fit build. We drank delicious green smoothies all week; I attended yoga daily and tried out barefoot running, which, combined with the power of green smoothies, gave me the leanest muscles I have ever had.

I credit the green smoothies to the fact that after losing 80 pounds I do not have any loose skin. Quite the opposite really, my skin was looking tighter, clearer, and younger than before. Along with looking great I felt great mentally; to be honest, I don't think I had even had a bad day the whole time I was on my health journey. I had completely reversed my PCOS and insulin issues; I was no longer anemic, and I was getting my period every twenty-nine days. My doctor was shocked but also excited for me; he could not believe his eyes after reading my blood tests.

I was so excited about my results both externally and internally that I started running classes on green smoothies and inspiring my friends, family, and clients to add green smoothies into their lives too and see and feel the benefits. I showed them how easy it is, even with a $30 blender. How they could make this delicious drink and either have one added into their existing diet or how they too could do their own smoothie retreat and only consume smoothies for a few days or a few weeks at home.

One time in 2012 I was doing a long green smoothie retreat at home. My partner and I had just moved to a new town, and to cope with stress during our relocation I wanted to let my body be filled with the healing powers of greens. On the forty-second day of drinking green smoothies for every meal, I suddenly started feeling queasy. At first, I thought my sickness came from cleaning up a house that had been unoccupied for over a year. When a girlfriend said to me "I bet you are pregnant," I replied, "No way. That is not possible; my partner and I have not been safe in seven years, and I have not even been close to falling pregnant." My friend insisted I take a pregnancy test, and to my shock I was!

During the first trimester I couldn't stomach green smoothies at all, but from the second trimester on I had one smoothie a day. I went forty-three weeks with my little bubba inside, nourishing both him and me with green smoothies. The midwives and obstetricians at the hospital were cranky at me for going so over and ran some tests. They were surprised to see that the cord, placenta, amniotic fluid, and baby were in perfect health. I labored for five days before my bubba decided to arrive. He came out with beautiful nourished skin, which surprised the midwife for such a full-term baby, but I am now getting used to being full of surprises, or should I say, green smoothies are full of surprises.

My little boy Finn is now eleven months old, and people comment on how clear his eyes are and how they sparkle. They are also surprised to see how lean and strong he is for such a young baby. He continued to have green smoothies through my breast milk and now we share a green smoothie every day. When Finn is given a piece of kale, he eats it and smiles. I even caught him today trying to eat the green part of the water melon. I call him "my little green head."

I cannot recommend green smoothies highly enough; they really did change my life!

Rebecca Wallis,
Sydney, Australia

TYPE 2 DIABETES REVERSED

I have attended many of Victoria's retreats over the years. The most memorable retreat for me was the retreat in Canada in 2009. During this retreat I met a family investigating alternative ways of healing their diabetes. I heard their personal story, which truly seemed to be a "medical miracle." Both an adult and a teenage young man were wearing insulin pumps twenty-four hours a day . . . but during this weeklong retreat they had to stop their pumps when their glucose went too low, and the insulin injections were no longer needed. Watching this happen firsthand is something I will always remember as a true "Green Smoothie Miracle."

I still drink green smoothies several times a week (basil, spinach, apple, and cayenne pepper are my favorite).

LM, Ashland, Oregon

KERRY, THE QUEEN OF GREENS FROM AUSTRALIA

Several years ago while looking for a way to improve my health I stumbled upon Victoria's website and green smoothies. Something resonated deep within me, as I was reading of the healing powers of chlorophyll that made a lot of sense.

At that time I knew I was eating and drinking too much processed junk food, too much fat, sugar, salt, and alcohol. I was feeling lethargic, overweight, unattractive, and depressed. I was feeding my body the wrong type of fuel and was running on empty.

I decided to start with what I was putting in my mouth. So I started making green smoothies and taking them to work, noticing a difference in how I was feeling very quickly. My mind and body were finally getting the nutrition they needed and craved. I started by replacing one meal a day with a liter of green smoothie. People began to take notice of this strange green concoction, which invited a lot of comments from the sublime to the ridiculous. Many were afraid to even try it.

I was having the last laugh here. I was experiencing many positive benefits from this simple formula. I felt happier, calmer, and had heaps more energy. I was losing weight and sleeping better. Naturally, I felt more confident and started to like myself! Soon people started noticing the changes in me and wanted to know more. My secret was out, and now everybody wanted to taste my green smoothie.

After a couple of years of experimenting with green smoothies I found myself eating more raw foods in general and reaping the benefits full time. And then a miracle happened. I received an email about Victoria soon coming to Australia to conduct her green smoothie retreat! I was beside myself, signing up immediately along with my sister and a friend, both of whom had never heard of Victoria Boutenko, let alone a green smoothie. Brave girls indeed because those seven days changed all our lives, and I haven't looked back since. In fact, I was so inspired I started a small business holding mini green smoothie retreats of my own here in Australia with many of my clients coming back a second and third time.

This is my green smoothie story that I hope will inspire, encourage, and motivate others to take up the green smoothie challenge and change their lives for the better too. It truly is one of the simplest, most inexpensive, and most important things that you can do for your general health and happiness.

Kerry Roberts, The Queen of Greens, Australia

THREE GENERATIONS BENEFITED
FROM GREEN SMOOTHIES

My journey started two years ago when I discovered a lump on my throat. The doctors said that it was a tumor, but didn't know if it was a malignant one. I started to read books that my mother gave me. But I didn't dare to trust that greens and organically grown food would take it away. I was afraid. So I had an operation and found out it was a benign tumor. After that I wanted to know more about greens and read books by Ann Wigmore and by Victoria Boutenko.

Since I participated in the green smoothie retreat in Sweden in 2013, I've been drinking green smoothies every day. I'm happy that I have persuaded my two children (two and six years of age) to drink a big green smoothie every morning. They love it and even ask for it! The smoothies disappear in two seconds. I don't know any other children who eat so many greens.

My benefits from the green smoothies are that my digestive tract works much better, and now I go to the bathroom once or twice a day. Before I went two times a week. I had eczema on my finger, but now it is gone! My skin is getting smoother, I have lost some weight, and when I work out I can exercise longer and at a higher pace. I have more energy and I am stronger!

My children are more alert and don't get tired as they did before. Also, their bowels work regularly. My oldest daughter used to cry from pain caused by constipation. Not anymore! Even my husband drinks green smoothies almost every day. As a family we consume a lot more vegetables than before. My next step is to inspire my dear friends to help themselves get better when they are ready.

Maria Larvall, Halmstad, Sweden

MY MOTHER'S STORY

About a year ago I found the book *Green for Life* by Victoria Boutenko. I bought it immediately. I have always had a great wish that I could make a green drink to get all the nutrition that I needed instead of spending hours by the stove cooking.

When I started reading the book, I understood that this was something extraordinary and bought a book for my daughter as well. Later she attended a retreat led by Victoria to learn more.

Nineteen years ago, when I was 52, I became hypersensitive to electromagnetic fields. At that time I was already hypersensitive to metals and chemicals. It has been a tough journey. I developed infections, which cause stiff joints and a general feeling of bad health, and I started taking antibiotics to manage inflammation. After every meal, I had severe pain on my right side—from gallstones—and I ate "stonebreaker pills" every day to feel good.

This summer I received a Vitamix blender as a birthday present from my children, and my daughter came to visit me and gave me some advice. I immediately started with green smoothies and felt that this was what I had been longing for, for so long!

Now I'm drinking green smoothies every day, combined with regular food. I've lost some weight, my colon is in better shape, and my gallstones are gone! I still take some antibiotics, but I feel that I'm getting my health back step by step.

I send my love to Victoria, my daughter Maria, my family, the chimpanzees and gorillas, and our wonderful green planet.

Iris Larvall, Sweden

IMPROVED VISION AND VIBRANT ENERGY

The green smoothie retreat in British Columbia in 2013 was a life-changing event for me as well as for my son once I got home and introduced this to him.

I have been drinking green smoothies since I met Victoria in Toronto at the Total Health Show in 2005. I was getting tired of having the same smoothies over and over again. Then I went to the retreat and learned tons of new information.

When I went to the retreat, I was not sure what to expect. We were served the smoothies and green soups, green puddings, and popsicles, along with lemon water.

Everyone around me was experiencing symptoms but not me. Then by the fourth day, I noticed I had canker sores in my mouth. This was very unusual for me. I also started to feel tired and a lack of energy. By the last day I was having difficulty with my vision. It seemed blurry and not in focus. I also felt a little foggy in the head. This was not my usual self as I usually had a clear head. However, after a couple of days, I got back to myself. I felt more alive than ever and with greater clarity. I was filled with a much higher energy level than I was accustomed to. Then my vision became clearer than it had been in the past. I now can see clearer and better with better focus.

I am able to deal with events in my life better than before. I want to fill my day with more adventures, planting more trees and plants for myself and my family; I am very enthusiastic about getting it all done in a short period of time. I want to be more sustainable.

Before the retreat, I stopped taking my herbal supplements and have not started taking them again. I understand better now that we are what we eat. When I give my body the nutrients that it needs, it sustains me and I am able to do anything that I desire to do.

That week on green smoothies has changed my life as well as the life of my special needs son. I will soon be coming out with a book on my son's journey.

Diane Braico, Lowbanks, Ontario, Canada

CANDIDA AND CHRONIC FATIGUE REVERSED

Following a positive diagnosis of malaria in 2009, I was left with a heavily compromised immune system. Candida was rampant; my body was a giant magnet for all viral and bacterial things. A chronic fatigue was starting to set in.

Desperate for change after having spent countless hours waiting in doctor's surgeries, consuming what I was prescribed with no effect at all, I reached the point of believing that there had to be another way.

At this time an invitation landed in my inbox from a friend of mine to attend Victoria, Sergei, and Valya's green smoothie retreat. I am a mother of two, and until the time of the retreat I had never attended a self-nurturing seminar like it before. Little did I know that it would change my life.

After giving my body a break by consuming nothing other than organic green smoothies for a week, I reached a point I never thought possible: not only did my body recover, my mind and spirit gained more and more clarity. The retreat allowed me to heal in a safe, holistic, loving, and nurturing environment.

Following the green smoothie retreat, I purchased a blender and set out to buy all things organic and green. After a few weeks my health continued to improve. The candida has not flared up since the retreat, the chronic fatigue and other ailments are a faint and distant memory, and the lack of medical bills speaks for itself. My life is now full of purpose and direction.

Green smoothies remain a constant in my family's life, as does the belief that our bodies are whole and complete. A number of friends and family were inspired by our family's transformation, and they too have embraced green smoothies into their lives. One friend rang me to apologize for having opposed my choice once he received the scientific evidence he needed from a TED talk by Dr. Terry Wahls. He too changed his diet, recovering from a number of autoimmune disorders.

JKM, Queensland, Australia

THE DOCTOR SAID, "WE WON'T SEE EACH OTHER ANYMORE."

When I was 26 years old, I became a victim of an incident and suffered from emotional damage. Soon I was also diagnosed with encephalitis (brain fever) and ankylosing spondylitis (AS), which is a form of inflammatory arthritis and caused a lot of pain for me. The doctors prescribed steroids and other medications to treat rheumatism. At that time I was a nurse, but I could not convince myself that the treatment would help me to get well, so I refused to take the treatment.

My health continued to decline.

One time, I noticed that the color of the white nurse robe I was wearing had turned blackish. I realized that my sweat was black. Even when I washed the robe, it would not come out, and I had to throw out a few of them. This shocking experience made me think seriously about detoxing, improving my bowel movements, and strengthening my natural immunity. The bowels have a deep connection with mental health; 95% of serotonin, which helps to maintain our mental balance, is primarily found in the gastrointestinal tract. So I tried to think of what would be good for the bowels.

I started to eat fresh food that gives more energy. I bought a blender and blended locally grown apples with native African greens called sukuma wiki, similar to kale, which is known for its high nutrition. Every morning I only drank this blend and water in order to detox. Now I know that this was a green smoothie.

Soon I noticed that I felt more energy and started to walk more than one hour every day and hike once a week (which I still do). Then I noticed something else had changed. While before I was emotionally depressed, now I felt love for small insects and worms, leaves and weeds that sway in the breeze, and realized that I am alive, thanks to nature. I felt appreciation. My mental health had improved, even better than when I used to be healthy.

Altogether I was sick and suffered for fourteen long years! I also had an articulation disorder, which resulted from the brain fever. I went through many rehabilitations. I experienced ureteric calculi, floating kidney, hydronephrosis, reflux esophagitis, gastritis, and constipation. I took some medications for ureteric calculi and constipation, but it was the green smoothies that cured all my ailments.

When I turned forty last year, I was thinking about my life and how I became sick and how I got well. I decided to tell as many people as I could about my experience with green smoothies. I attended a Green Smoothie Workshop and learned many helpful tips for smoothie making. I was very impressed at how good green smoothies tasted. I feel so happy every day when I make my smoothies.

After that I started drinking a lot more green smoothies than before. I noticed that the pain in my lower back had almost gone away. A little while ago I went to the hospital to check up on my AS. The doctor told me I no longer had AS. It was cured. The doctor asked me if I had done something special, and I told him about green smoothies. He wrote a note and said, "We won't see each other anymore." Then he congratulated me. I was very pleasantly surprised!

On the train on the way home, I was thinking that my body was really no longer in any pain or suffering any other inconvenience.

Healthy bowels are the key to a healthy mind and body. I am confident that drinking green smoothies is the correct way to detox. I am thankful to Victoria Boutenko for green smoothies and for their introduction in Japan. My wish is to accurately teach about green smoothies in Japan.

Sumie Yoshino, Gunma Prefecture, Japan

GREEN SMOOTHIES ARE SATIATING

I was only vaguely familiar with green smoothies before I went to the retreat on Vancouver Island in August of 2009; I had no health expectations going to the retreat except for a bit of dread about eating only green smoothies for a week: Would I starve to death? Hilarious now that I say that.

Instead of being weak with starvation, I felt more energy than I'd experienced in years, and I was never hungry. I know I slept more soundly and felt stronger and more mentally clear when I left than when I arrived.

I remember a man at our retreat who was diabetic and how we collectively watched him transform over the week. By the time we left, he literally looked ten years younger and had significantly reduced his insulin intake!

The first thing I did when I got home was buy a Vitamix. Even after all these years, I still start every morning with a green smoothie that I prepare the night before. I think living for seven days on green smoothies started a habit for me. I don't know if I would have continued with the green smoothies if I had only tried them in a one-day workshop. I started out with the recipes I learned at the retreat and from the book *Green Smoothie Revolution,* but now I mostly wing it with whatever greens/fruits I have in the fridge; they always taste great.

Dian Quinney, Calgary, Alberta, Canada

SEVEN DAYS OF GREEN MAGIC

My name is Edda, and I live in Iceland. I attended two retreats with Victoria in Sweden in 2011 and in 2013. On my first stay I learned so much that I wanted to reinforce my knowledge by participating again.

All I did was eat these green smoothies and enjoy yoga and sunshine every morning and lectures during the day. We also drank a lot of water with lemon slices. This food had a massive effect on all of us. During the first two days all of us in the group started experiencing a wide variety of detox symptoms. I had a lot of mucus in my throat most of the week and headache in the back of my head. Everybody in the group was detoxing during the first days, but by the end of the week we all felt so good that we could not take the smile off our faces.

In only a week we changed dramatically. I felt so wonderful that I threw away my medicines. I especially liked going out in the field and picking wild greens with Victoria's son Sergei and learning how easy it was to get good food for nothing.

Since this retreat I have been enjoying green smoothies every morning, and my body craves them. They have become the foundation for my health. I like to prepare for myself a fresh one every morning, not less than a liter. My dream is to teach a lot of people here in Iceland to drink green smoothies every day because of the amazing health benefits they give you and the joy of picking your own greens in nature.

Edda, Iceland

TEACHER INSPIRED STUDENTS TO DRINK GREEN SMOOTHIES

In 2010, I decided to join the Boutenko family and others for the retreat in Queensland, Australia. I was deeply impressed with what I learned, especially the positive changes in people with cancer and diabetes.

I understand the healing powers of green smoothies and how they heal. When I returned from the retreat, I continued with the smoothies for many more weeks to overcome the removal of amalgam from my teeth, and I am convinced it helped me through the detox period.

I am a teacher, who gets to class with a green drink, and my students have been curious and willing to try. There have been a few who even adapted to drinking green smoothies! As soon as I am able to, I want to attend another retreat and experience the cleansing and calming effect the green smoothie retreat had on me.

Eva, Australia

STOMACH PAINS COMPLETELY GONE

In 2011 I talked my now husband into attending the Boutenko family green smoothie retreat in New South Wales, Australia. It was one of the biggest and best challenges I have done in my life. It is a time that I reflect on often, which gives me inspiration to continue the journey of striving for better health.

While I didn't have the major health concerns that many people are facing today, such as cancers or diabetes, I suffered for about two years with overpowering pains in my stomach and had no idea why I had them. I was confused for a long time considering that I was eating a "healthy" diet: salad, sandwiches, rolls, breakfast cereals, pastas, rice. All the while I was complaining every day about the pains in my stomach, and most days I would have to lie down to try to "stretch" out the pain and wait until it went away. My husband borrowed a book from our local library written by two kids, Valya and Sergei Boutenko. He started talking to me about and making the raw foods and green smoothies that these two kids had written about. I remember my very first green smoothie—mango, banana, and spinach—delicious! Gradually I swapped my cereal to green smoothies for breakfast. Once we started, we noticed that the pains in my stomach were not as bad.

At the end of 2010 I heard about the retreat that Victoria, Valya, and Sergei were hosting in Australia in April of 2011. I begged my husband to go; we took time off from work and flew to New South Wales for the seven-day retreat. This was a life-changing experience for us. When we returned, we bought a Vitamix blender and have used it every day at least twice a day! Now I have had a baby, and she too drinks green smoothies!

During the retreat we drank *only* green smoothies from morning until night and as much as we wanted. On day two I wondered if I was going to make it through the week. We woke up every morning by 5:30–6:00 a.m. and started our day with a choice of barefoot running or yoga. By day three I recognized that I was waking up feeling refreshed and with a lot of energy and was surprised that I did not feel tired. After our morning exercise we drank a glass of green smoothie (or two or three) while sitting around with the other people participating in the retreat. We met some very interesting people, most who were there because of health issues they had. We talked about our journey with green smoothies, health issues, swapped ideas, and one lady even gave us her "travel blender" so we could continue drinking green smoothies on our extended holiday after the retreat finished! During the days we watched Valya demonstrating how to make the perfect smoothie, we listened to Victoria on her research into green smoothies, we picked wild edibles with Sergei, and we had time to ourselves to wander around the beautiful grounds if we wanted. At night we watched documentaries on a range of health issues, which were informative and also life changing. During the week my body showed signs of detoxing (headaches, cramps, etc.), and I remember Victoria saying to embrace these feelings. I now understand that it was my body getting rid of all the "garbage" and that I needed to go through this process.

By day seven I felt energetic, light, my stomach felt great, and I felt a huge sense of achievement. I would be travelling for another three weeks after the retreat finished and wanted this feeling to last so I knew that I had to continue drinking green smoothies. Thank goodness for the travel blender! I'll never forget my first "foods" that I ate at the airport after leaving the retreat.

Still to this very day, my husband and I, and now my nine-month-old baby, drink a green smoothie every day. Some of our families and friends have now too incorporated green smoothies into their daily lives. I do not get any pains anymore in my stomach unless I eat something that I know I shouldn't. It has been nearly four years now.

Carmen Moyse, Adelaide, Australia

I FEEL YOUNGER, HEALTHIER, AND HAPPIER THAN EVER

When I was a kid, the hospitals were my second home. Respiratory system diseases like pneumonia, bronchitis, tonsillitis, cold, and flu had been accompanying me my entire childhood and youth. Two times I had nearly died from suffocation. Aggressive treatment with strong and multiple antibiotics and steroids made me sick further, severely damaging my immune and digestive systems. At twenty I felt like a very old person: weak, pale, exhausted, miserable, and scared for my future. Nothing was interesting to me; I had a bloated stomach, severe constipation, fatigue, poor sleep, high blood pressure, and declined memory and cognitive function.

After I came across green smoothies, my life improved dramatically. Gradually, all diseases started to disappear. Green smoothies nourished not only my body but my mind and soul as well. My immune system exploded with strength; my energy level has boosted rapidly. All negative emotions that I used to have, such as bad mood, fear, nervousness, and depression, vanished. My self-esteem and self-confidence levels have risen. I turned into a determined and motivated person. My relationship with family, friends, and myself became friendly and positive. My attitude toward other people and society became spiritual, peaceful, and conscious. My career and financial well-being acquired strict outlines. I was able to design a new, clear intention and goal for my life.

My digestive problems have been completely solved: a stool of two to three times a day has become a common feature, there is no more heavy, bloated feeling in my gut, and my weight is now stable.

I completely forgot about any respiratory problems, such as a cold, flu, sore throat, and so on. I don't feel any more lack of energy, exhaustion, and hypertension; my skin now is shiny and bright. I look and feel younger, better, and happier than ever.

Igor P-k, Chicago, Illinois

OUT OF THE WHEELCHAIR
AND RHEUMATOID ARTHRITIS GONE

During a trip to Los Angeles, I stayed with close friends who are sisters. One of the sisters was confined to a wheelchair. She had spent almost a year being bedridden and needed constant care by her live-in housekeeper.

One day, I purchased a high-powered blender to give to my friends and eagerly demonstrated how to make green smoothies thinking it might become a part of their daily ritual. One of the sisters, Christine, readily consumed it while the wheelchair-bound sister, Celeste, politely sipped it, said it tasted okay, and then put it down, saying she'd already eaten.

Undaunted, I left the blender and the ingredients for their housekeeper to keep providing them with green smoothies while I was away. I was greatly disappointed when I received a message from them that the blender was packed up and ready to be taken with me the next time I visited.

However, a few weeks later I was shocked when I received another message that Celeste had changed her mind. Apparently, her housekeeper enjoyed the green smoothies and had been making them for herself. Celeste was impressed with all the significant improvements in her housekeeper's appearance, such as weight loss, higher energy level, positive attitude, and so on. She wondered what her secret was.

"Green smoothies!" her housekeeper gladly shared. So the next time I visited I was greeted by happy and positive remarks by Celeste who had previously dismissed the green smoothies as unimportant.

But that was just the beginning! The next time I visited, my friend was out of her wheelchair, walking around easily, happy as a lark, and even out driving and taking short trips by herself. Additionally, this mother, grandmother, and great-grandmother took great pleasure sharing her newly discovered "elixir" with everyone she met.

Celeste now often invites her grandchildren and great-grandchildren into the kitchen and personally shows them how to make green smoothies.

Gerry Coffey, Decatur, Alabama

ADDITIONAL LETTER FROM CHRISTINE

Dear Gerry,

The events just happened six days ago. At times I was only 90% sure it was only the green smoothies that cured Celeste, as she was taking prescription medication for her crippling rheumatoid arthritis. One day she cut out the medication without telling the doctor, depending only on green smoothies and was completely healed, saying that she felt like she was twenty-five years young.

Celeste has been consuming green smoothies daily and has been free of rheumatoid arthritis for more than two years. But then, unfortunately, she cut back on the smoothies, drinking them only once a week. As a consequence, last week she had a flare-up of her rheumatoid arthritis, swelling of the left wrist and hand, nausea; she felt horrible. This time she went to a doctor, who verified it was rheumatoid arthritis and recommended a drug to take and a pain medicine.

Celeste, in her wisdom, refused the doctor's advice on both counts. She knew she could overcome the flare-up with green smoothies. She began drinking them again every day, stopped eating inflammatory foods, and I am very happy to report that all symptoms are gone; she feels great and is looking forward to the future, all thanks to green smoothies. Without a shadow of a doubt, it's the green smoothies that keep the rheumatoid arthritis away.

Celeste has been a constant promoter of Victoria's recipes among her friends. For example, her dear friend, who is ninety years old, swears by his daily intake, which keeps him free of arthritis and the aches and pains that his roommate endures. And her children, grandchildren, and six great-grandchildren all drink smoothies daily, thanks to our friend Gerry who gave us the right machine.

How blessed we are to have found this great secret to good health. If only the world would listen!

Christine

FROM MOM TO DAUGHTER TO FAMILY TO ALL PEOPLE OF SEATTLE: DRINK SMOOTHIES!

My mom has always been an explorer. During the summer of 2010 she attended her first green smoothie retreat with the Boutenkos. When she returned home, she was radiant and inspired. She had lost over ten pounds, and her skin was glowing. She couldn't stop talking about green smoothies and immediately bought a Vitamix for our family home.

I was slightly skeptical of her enthusiasm. Was this just another one of her crazy fads that would fade in a few months? Luckily her persistence persuaded me and the rest of the family to try her latest discovery. After listening to her testimony of weight loss and increased energy I decided to give the green drink a try. Green smoothies became a part of my life, but on a diminutive scale for about a year. I drank green smoothies when my mom made them for me and once in a while made my own. A year later my mom was still inspired about smoothies and asked me to attend a retreat with her in Canada.

In August 2011 I attended the green smoothie retreat. It combined drinking green smoothies with workshops and exercise. I attended the retreat with my mom and sister. For seven days we consumed four green smoothies a day along with raw vegetables. Attending the retreat had a hugely positive impact on my life. During the retreat I saw the benefits of green smoothies immediately manifest in my body. My skin, hair, and nails all became stronger and softer. My appetite decreased, and I realized that my body requires less food than I was taking in, as long as I was eating nutritious, raw, whole foods. I lost seven pounds in the seven-day retreat and felt much lighter and less toxic.

Before attending the retreat I was apprehensive about only consuming green smoothies, raw fruits, and vegetable for seven long days, without a normal meal. I love food and didn't think it would be possible for me. After the first two days that apprehension had disappeared. Now almost three years later I am still consuming green smoothies daily and talking about them to anyone who will listen. I bring my mason jar filled with different colored green smoothies to my nanny job, to yoga, and anywhere else I go in my daily life. Even the boys that I nanny, ages three and one, are in love with green smoothies. I always have to bring an extra big jar so that I can share my smoothies with them. Through their love of smoothies their parents even decided to buy a Vitamix and started blending up amazing green drinks themselves. The little boys fell in love with smoothies, which also helped with keeping the boys pooping normally.

My entire family of eight, drinks green smoothies, and we share them with everyone who visits our home. Many of my friends have purchased blenders and have asked me to share tips and recipes for making smoothies. My friends all rave about how much more energy they have when they drink their greens.

I am so passionate about green smoothies that I am currently working to create my own green smoothie business so that I can spread my love of green smoothies and health to more people in Seattle.

Stephanie Brossmann, Seattle, Washington

SOMETIMES IT TAKES LONGER TO HEAL

I had an unusual experience in that I didn't feel better during the retreat. People around me were excited and thriving, and I was constipated and fuzzy-headed. But I took to heart what I was learning about green smoothies. I went home, bought a blender, watched the DVDs, and loaded up on raw fruits and vegetables.

I was not a miracle case in that I did not heal overnight. I transformed over weeks and months. However, I did heal! The irritable bowel syndrome was gone. My sinuses cleared up. I lost 25 pounds. My energy is now fantastic.

I have incorporated other foods into my dining now, but a green smoothie each day is a must. When I travel and am unable to make green smoothies, I can tell that my body misses them. And certainly when I am sick, I revert back to an all green smoothie diet.

The retreat taught me a way of life that gives me more choices. It was necessary for me to learn at a retreat because of the support a retreat affords. Reading a book doesn't cut it when considering life changes.

Cindy Patterson, Ashland, Oregon

MOM PUT SON'S HIGH SCHOOL ON GREEN SMOOTHIES FOR A YEAR

My name is Isabelle, and I went to the retreat because I read Victoria Boutenko's book *Green for Life*. When I learned she was having a week of green smoothies, I jumped on it for the adventure. Having a whole week of green smoothies was transformational for me. I liked the first retreat so much that I came to participate a second time.

First of all and that might seem trivial to you, I felt a tightening of the skin in my face as if I was getting younger and more vital. Before I went to the retreat, I was suffering heavily from depression almost every day, and, if I skipped my medication for one day, I felt terrible in the afternoon. When I was at the retreat, I noticed I forgot about taking my medications for two or three days, and I felt incredibly light and happy.

My doctor realized that after the retreat I felt the best she has ever seen me. Now when I am not feeling well, my doctor asks me what I have been eating. She recommends me to have green smoothies and some raw food every day.

I was very inspired after that workshop, and I made green smoothies for all the kids in my son's high school. Students and teachers loved it and were curious what that green stuff was. Encouraged, I made it once a week for a year for all one hundred students of this high school. I got a reputation at school as "the green smoothie lady."

However, the next year the number of students went up to two hundred, and I could not keep it up anymore. I was touched when a lot of students asked me the next year, "What about the green smoothies?" I encouraged them to make smoothies themselves because every time I served them smoothies, I wrote the recipe on a big board. One time, three years later, I found myself sitting next to one student at the movie theater and she told me, "Your smoothies were good. I miss them." I was moved that I was able to touch that generation of teenagers that in general were more interested in fast food than any healthy stuff. My son is in a faraway college now, but whenever a friend from his high school came over to our house, he was offered a green smoothie and appreciated it.

I am still very good at making green smoothies like this very simple one: spinach, very ripe pears, and ginger. It is a winner every time. Enjoy your green smoothies!

Isabelle, Redwood City, California

PART THREE

Recipes

SWEET GREEN SMOOTHIES

ORIGINAL RAW FAMILY SMOOTHIE

YIELDS 2 QUARTS

1 bunch (3 cups) spinach
2 cups strawberries (fresh or frozen)
2 ripe bananas
2 cups water

BLACKBERRY STRENGTH

YIELDS 2 QUARTS

1 pint blackberries
1 ripe mango, in chunks
3 cups red kale, stems removed
2 cups water

TROPICAL VIGOR

YIELDS 2 QUARTS

1 cup pineapple chunks
1 cup mango chunks
1 banana
½ bunch Swiss chard, stems removed
2 cups water

RASPBERRY KOMBUCHA CRUSH

YIELDS 2 QUARTS

2 cups kale, stems removed

1 cup raspberries

1 mango, in chunks

2 cups kombucha

SWEET EMERALD

YIELDS 2 QUARTS

2 cups grapes (seedless)

3 kiwis, peeled

2 bananas

½ bunch red leaf lettuce

2 cups water

SUPER GREEN MISSION

YIELDS 2 QUARTS

2 cups kale, stems removed

1 organic cucumber, with peel

3 ripe pears, in chunks without cores

1 lime, juiced

2 cups water

PARSLEY ENTHUSIASM

YIELDS 2 QUARTS

1 bunch fresh parsley

2 kiwis, peeled

1 apple, cut up without core

1 ripe banana

2 cups kombucha

TWIRLING DANDELION

YIELDS 2 QUARTS

3 cups dandelion greens

2 ripe mangos, in chunks

1 cup apple juice

1 cup water

ABSOLUTELY PEACHY

YIELDS 2 QUARTS

5 peaches, without pits

1 head butterhead lettuce

2 cups water

DANDELION WINE

YIELDS 2 QUARTS

1 bunch dandelion greens

2 mangos, in chunks

3 cups apple juice

1 cup water

WATERMELON FRESHNESS

YIELDS 2 QUARTS

5 cups fresh watermelon chunks, **rind removed**

1 banana

2 cups baby spinach

½ lemon, juiced

EMERALD PAPAYA

YIELDS 2 QUARTS

3 cups spinach

2 fresh papayas, peeled with **seeds removed**

1 banana

2 cups water

SWEET GREEN MELON

YIELDS 2 QUARTS

5 cups cantaloupe cubes

2 cups green leaf lettuce

½ cup cranberries (fresh or frozen)

1 cup water

GREEN GIFT FOR KIDNEYS

YIELDS 2 QUARTS

5 cups cantaloupe cubes

1 bunch fresh parsley

½ lime, with peel

DELICIOUS SURPRISE

YIELDS 2 QUARTS

1 head butterhead lettuce

1 apple, cut up without core

1 ripe orange, peeled with seeds removed

1 cup strawberries

2 cups water

LOVELY GREEN GOODNESS

YIELDS 2 QUARTS

3 cups green oak leaf lettuce

2 bananas

1 apple, cut up without core

1 pear, in chunks without core

2 cups water

MINTY DELICACY

YIELDS 2 QUARTS

2 cups pineapple chunks

1 cup mango chunks

1 banana

½ bunch kale, stems removed

1 sprig mint

2 cups water

SWEET PARSLEY

YIELDS 2 QUARTS

2 cups parsley

1 apple, cut up without core

1 banana

2 Medjool dates, without pits

½ lime, with peel

GREEN LIFT

YIELDS 2 QUARTS

3 cups romaine lettuce

1 mango, in chunks

1 cup blueberries

1 small piece gingerroot

2 cups water

IMMUNITY STRENGTHENER

YIELDS 2 QUARTS

2 cups spinach

1 cup arugula

1 apple, cut up without core

1 banana

½ cup cranberries (fresh or frozen)

2 cups water

GREEN SOUPS

These two blends are to be used to add spice to other soup recipies.

🐝 SUPER SPICY GARLIC BLEND

YIELDS 1 QUART

½ avocado

½ cup garlic cloves

1 lemon (juiced with seeds removed)

3 cups water

🐝 SUPER SPICY PEPPER BLEND

YIELDS 1 QUART

½ avocado

4 jalapeno peppers

1 lemon (juiced with seeds removed)

3 cups water

GREEN CHOWDER

YIELDS 2 QUARTS

2 cups spinach

2 cups arugula

1 cup cherry tomatoes

½ bunch fresh dill (or any other herb you can find)

2 stalks celery

1 avocado

2 limes, juiced

2 cups water

PEPPERS AND TOMATOES

YIELDS 2 QUARTS

3 cups baby spinach

3 red bell peppers

3 ripe tomatoes

1 avocado

½ bunch basil

1 lime, juiced

2 cups water

SPICY FRESHNESS

YIELDS 2 QUARTS

1 cup mustard leaves

1 avocado

2 cucumbers, with peel

½ bunch cilantro

1 lemon, juiced, seeds removed

2 cups water

ITALIAN SOUP

YIELDS 2 QUARTS

3 cups spinach

3 stalks celery

½ cup basil

1 red bell pepper

1 ripe tomato

1 avocado

½ jalapeño pepper

2 limes, juiced

2 cups water

GAZPACHO

YIELDS 2 QUARTS

3 leaves kale, stems removed

1 bunch basil

3 large tomatoes

2 stalks celery

1 red bell pepper

1 avocado

2 limes, juiced

1 clove garlic

2 cups water

THAI SOUP

YIELDS 2 QUARTS

6 leaves kale, stems removed

2 cucumbers, with peel

1 avocado

2 limes, juiced

3 cloves garlic

½ inch fresh turmeric root (or ½ teaspoon powdered turmeric)

½ inch fresh gingerroot (or ¼ teaspoon dried ground ginger)

2 cups water

CUCUMBER DILL SOUP

YIELDS 2 QUARTS

2 cucumbers, with peel

½ bunch dill

1 avocado

5 leaves chard, stems removed

2 stalks celery

2 limes, juiced

2 cloves garlic

2 cups water

HERB GARDEN

YIELDS 2 QUARTS

5 leaves chard, stems removed

1 sprig oregano

1 sprig rosemary

1 sprig parsley

1 avocado

2 cucumbers, with peel

2 limes, juiced

2 cups water

SPICY AND SOUR TOMATO SOUP

YIELDS 2 QUARTS

1 bunch watercress

½ bunch basil

5 large ripe tomatoes

1 avocado

2 lemons, juiced with seeds removed

2 cups water

CREAM OF SPROUTS

YIELDS 2 QUARTS

2 cups sunflower sprouts

½ cup parsley

½ cup dill

1 cucumber, with peel

2 tomatoes

1 avocado

2 lemons, juiced with seeds removed

2 cups water

SPICY GREEN SOUP

YIELDS 2 QUARTS

2 cups radish tops
½ cup fresh basil
1 avocado
2 red bell peppers
2 limes, peeled
2 cups water

DANDELION SOUP

YIELDS 2 QUARTS

1 cup dandelion greens
1 cup chard, stems removed
2 stalks celery
1 avocado
2 cucumbers, with peel
4 limes, juiced
1 small piece gingerroot
2 cups water

GREEN PUDDINGS

MANGO ECSTASY

YIELDS 3 CUPS

1 bunch chard, stems removed

2 mangos, in chunks

1 pear, in chunks without core

1 banana

SWEET BITE

YIELDS 3 CUPS

7 leaves kale, stems removed

4 pears, in chunks without cores

1 banana

½ lime, with peel

1 pinch of cayenne

THE PROOF IS IN THIS PUDDING

YIELDS 3 CUPS

1 bunch parsley

2 cups pineapple chunks

1 mango, in chunks

1 ripe orange, peeled with seeds removed

PERSIMMON PUDDING

YIELDS 3 CUPS

5 persimmons, peeled with seeds removed

3 cups baby spinach

1 ripe banana

½ lime, with peel

NECTAR VERDE

YIELDS 3 CUPS

1 Mexican papaya, peeled with seeds removed

1 cup spinach

½ lime, with peel

1 teaspoon chia seeds

GLORIOUS SPROUTS

YIELDS 3 CUPS

1 cup sunflower sprouts

4 peaches, pits removed

1 apple, cut up without core

1 lime, juiced

SMOOTH MELON

YIELDS 3 CUPS

2 cups green leaf lettuce
½ honeydew melon, in cubes
1 mango, in chunks
1 lime, juiced

PINK ELEGANCE

YIELDS 3 CUPS

2 cups beet greens
1 cup cranberries (fresh or frozen)
5 Medjool dates, without pits
1 banana
1 orange, peeled with seeds removed
1 teaspoon chia seeds

MINTY LEMON DESSERT

YIELDS 3 CUPS

1 cup spinach
1 banana
2 mangos, in chunks
1 orange, peeled with seeds removed
1 lemon, peeled with seeds removed
1 sprig mint
1 teaspoon psyllium husk powder

PINK COCONUT

YIELDS 3 CUPS

2 cups romaine lettuce

1 young coconut, water and meat included

2 cups strawberries

1 lemon, peeled with seeds removed

MANGO JOY

YIELDS 3 CUPS

½ bunch chard, stems removed

3 mangos, in chunks

1 cup cranberries

EMERALD APPLESAUCE

YIELDS 3 CUPS

4 apples, cut up without cores

1 banana

2 cups spinach

½ teaspoon cinnamon

1 cup water

BEST PUDDING

YIELDS 3 CUPS

2 mangos, in chunks
2 cups Swiss chard, stems removed
1 cup pineapple chunks
½ lime, with peel

PURPLE VITALITY

YIELDS 3 CUPS

1 cup dandelion greens
2 cups blueberries
1 orange, peeled with seeds removed
1 small piece gingerroot

KIWI DESSERT

YIELDS 3 CUPS

5 leaves kale, stems removed
2 stalks celery
1 cup pineapple chunks
1 banana
4 ripe kiwis, peeled
1 teaspoon psyllium husk powder

GREEN DREAM POPSICLES

YIELDS 2 QUARTS (6 TO 10 POPSICLES, DEPENDING ON SIZE OF MOLDS)

2 cups spinach

2 cups raspberries

1 cup cranberries

2 bananas

5 Medjool dates, without pits

1 teaspoon psyllium husk powder

1 cup water

Blend all ingredients well, pour into popsicle holders, and freeze.

LAYERED GREEN PUDDING

YIELDS 10 CUPS

This elegant green smoothie looks and tastes perfect for the holiday season. We serve it at all our retreats, and it has become one of our most popular smoothies.

Put 10 clear glasses on a tray.
For the bottom layer, blend the following ingredients well:

    1 cup blackberries
    2 apples, cut up without cores
    1 lemon, sliced with peel on
    4 sprigs mint
    2 cups water

The liquid in your blender will be thin. Set your blender to a lower speed, and add four heaping teaspoons of psyllium husk powder while the blender is running. Stop the blender, and quickly pour the liquid into the glasses, filling each glass approximately one-third.

For the middle layer, blend the following ingredients well:

    4 cups spinach (or 1 bunch)
    2 ripe bananas
    3 oranges, peeled and sliced with seeds removed
    2 cups water

The liquid in your blender will be thin. Set your blender to a lower speed, and add four heaping teaspoons of psyllium husk powder while the blender is running. Stop the blender, and quickly pour the liquid into the glasses, filling each glass approximately one-third, on top of the bottom layer.

For the top layer, blend the following ingredients well:

2 cups cranberries
7 large dates, without pits
1 ripe banana
2 cups water

The liquid in your blender will be thin. Set your blender to a lower speed, and add four heaping teaspoons of psyllium husk powder while the blender is running. Stop the blender, and quickly pour the liquid into the glasses, over the two previous layers. The pudding will solidify in a matter of minutes. Decorate with fresh fruit, berries, and greens.

SALADS AND SOUPS POPULAR IN MY FAMILY

I invite you to use these healthy recipes for some of your meals after you finish your seven-day green smoothie retreat. Use them as basic ideas and try creating your own salads and soups.

A SATISFYING SALAD

SERVES 3

5 cups baby greens, chopped
1 carrot, grated
¼ daikon radish, grated
1 cucumber, chopped
5 green onions, chopped
½ bunch fresh basil, chopped
4 tablespoons nutritional yeast
3 tablespoons salsa
1 tablespoon oil
¼ teaspoon salt (optional)

Mix all the ingredients together in a large bowl, and serve.

WEIGHT-LOSS SALAD

SERVES 2

1 sweet potato, peeled and steamed
2 cups celery, finely chopped
2 cucumbers, sliced
¼ teaspoon salt
2 cloves fresh garlic, chopped
¼ teaspoon cayenne pepper

In a large bowl, use a fork to mash the sweet potato. Add the remaining ingredients, mix together, and serve.

RUSSIAN SALAD "VINAIGRETTE"

SERVES 3

1 bunch fresh arugula

1 raw beet, peeled

1 raw carrot, peeled

½ apple, grated

2 pickles, sliced

½ avocado, in chunks

1 red onion, sliced

4 sprigs dill weed, chopped

1 cup frozen peas

½ orange, juiced

1 tablespoon olive oil

½ teaspoon sea salt

Wash the arugula in a large bowl of water so that any particles of dirt sink to the bottom of the bowl and do not end up in your salad. Chop the arugula and place it in a salad bowl. Grate the beet, carrot, and apple on top of the arugula. Add the pickles, avocado, onion, and dill weed. Place the peas in a small pot and fill it with water. Bring the water to a boil, then immediately drain the water and mix the peas in with the rest of the ingredients. Pour the orange juice and oil over the salad, and serve sprinkled with the salt.

MICRO SPROUT SALAD

SERVES 2

6 cups microgreens
4 green onions, chopped
¼ teaspoon salt
1 tablespoon olive oil
3 tablespoons nutritional yeast

Mix ingredients thoroughly in a large bowl, and serve.

TURNIP SALAD

SERVES 2

2 turnips, grated
1 carrot, grated
4 green onions, chopped
1 bunch cilantro, chopped
1 medium tomato, chopped
2 cloves fresh garlic, minced
½ teaspoon salt
1 tablespoon olive oil

Mix all the ingredients together in a large bowl, and serve.

CABBAGE SALAD

¼ cabbage, chopped

1 red bell pepper, chopped

5 sprigs parsley, chopped

3 green onions, chopped

1 tablespoon olive oil

2 tablespoons nutritional yeast

½ lemon, juiced

¼ teaspoon salt

Mix all the ingredients together in a large bowl, and serve.

LENTILS WITH VEGGIES SOUP

SERVES 3

4 cups water

2 cups lentils, soaked overnight

1 medium sweet potato, peeled and cubed

1 red bell pepper, chopped

2 stalks celery, chopped

5 large cloves garlic, peeled and chopped

½ teaspoon cayenne pepper

½ teaspoon salt

3 tablespoons lemon juice

1 green onion, diced

1 sprig fresh dill weed

Bring the water to a boil in a stockpot, and then add the lentils. Stir immediately to keep the lentils from sticking to the bottom of the pan. After 15 minutes, add the rest of the ingredients except for the lemon juice, green onion, and dill weed. Continue cooking for 10 more minutes at a low boil or until the potatoes are done. Turn off the heat, and add the lemon juice. Serve sprinkled with the green onions and dill weed.

BOK CHOY SOUP

SERVES 3

4 cups water

1 medium sweet potato, peeled and cubed

1 carrot, julienned

2 cups broccoli florets

5 baby bok choy stalks, chopped

5 button or cremini mushrooms, chopped

2 medium tomatoes, chopped

½ teaspoon salt

½ teaspoon cayenne pepper

3 tablespoons lemon juice

1 tablespoon olive oil (optional)

1 sprig parsley or other fresh herbs, diced

Bring the water to a boil in a stockpot. Add the sweet potato, carrot, and broccoli, stirring immediately to keep the veggies from sticking to the bottom of the pan. After 5 minutes, add the bok choy, mushrooms, and tomatoes. Continue cooking for 3 more minutes at a low boil. Turn off the heat, and add the salt, cayenne pepper, lemon juice, and olive oil. Serve sprinkled with the parsley.

BEET SOUP

4 cups water

2 medium beets, peeled and cubed

¼ cabbage, chopped

1 carrot, julienned

1 potato, peeled and diced

1 inch gingerroot, sliced

1 onion, diced

3 cups stinging nettles (or spinach), chopped

½ teaspoon salt

3 tablespoons lemon juice

1 tablespoon olive oil (optional)

1 sprig parsley or other fresh herbs, diced

Bring the water to a boil in a stockpot, and then add the beets. Stir immediately to keep the beets from sticking to the bottom of the pan. After 15 minutes, add the cabbage, carrot, potato, gingerroot, and onion. Continue cooking for 5 more minutes at a low boil. Add the nettles, and continue cooking at a low boil for 3 more minutes. Turn off the heat and add the salt, lemon juice, and olive oil. Serve sprinkled with the parsley.

CREAM OF BROCCOLI SOUP

SERVES 3

4 cups water

1 medium sweet potato, peeled and cubed

1 medium potato, peeled and diced

5 cups broccoli, chopped

2 medium tomatoes, chopped

5 sprigs basil, chopped

½ teaspoon salt

½ teaspoon cayenne pepper

3 tablespoons lemon juice

1 tablespoon olive oil (optional)

1 sprig parsley or other fresh herbs, diced

Bring the water to a boil in a stockpot, and then add the potatoes. Stir immediately to keep the potatoes from sticking to the bottom of the pan. After 5 minutes, add the broccoli, tomatoes, and basil. Continue cooking for 5 more minutes at a low boil. Turn off the heat, and add the salt, cayenne pepper, lemon juice, and olive oil. Serve sprinkled with the parsley.

CREAM OF NETTLES SOUP

4 cups water

2 medium sweet potatoes, peeled and cubed

3 cups stinging nettles (or spinach), chopped

2 stalks celery, chopped

5 sprigs cilantro, chopped

½ cup rolled oats

½ teaspoon cayenne pepper

½ teaspoon salt

3 tablespoons lemon juice

1 tablespoon olive oil (optional)

1 sprig parsley or other fresh herbs, diced

Bring the water to a boil in a stockpot, and then add the sweet potatoes. Stir immediately to keep the potatoes from sticking to the bottom of the pan. After 5 minutes, add the nettles, celery, cilantro, oats, and cayenne pepper. Continue cooking for 3 more minutes at a low boil. Turn off the heat, and add the salt, lemon juice, and olive oil. Serve sprinkled with the parsley.

BIBLIOGRAPHY

Anderson, Mike. *Healing Cancer from Inside Out.* DVD. Directed by Mike Anderson. Glendale, CA: RaveDiet.com, 2009.

Boutenko, Sergei. *Wild Edibles.* Berkeley, CA: North Atlantic Books, 2013.

Boutenko, Sergei, and Valya Boutenko. *Fresh: The Ultimate Live-Food Cookbook.* Berkeley, CA: North Atlantic Books, 2008.

Boutenko, Victoria. *Green for Life.* Berkeley, CA: North Atlantic Books, 2010.

——. *Green Smoothie Revolution.* Berkeley, CA: North Atlantic Books, 2009.

——. *12 Steps to Raw Foods.* Berkeley, CA: North Atlantic Books, 2007.

Bragg, Paul, and Patricia Bragg. *The Shocking Truth about Water.* Santa Barbara, CA: Health Science Publications, 1985.

Campbell, T. Colin. *The China Study.* Dallas, TX: BenBella Books, 2006.

Chopra, Deepak. *Perfect Health: The Complete Mind Body.* New York, NY: Three Rivers Press, 2001.

Dean, Carolyn. *The Magnesium Miracle.* New York, NY: Ballantine Books, 2006.

Ehret, Arnold. *Rational Fasting: Regeneration Diet and Natural Cure for All Diseases.* New York, NY: Ehret Literature, 2011.

Fuhrman, Joel. *Eat to Live: The Revolutionary Formula for Fast and Sustained Weight Loss.* New York, NY: Little, Brown and Company, 2011.

Jensen, Bernard. *Come Alive!* San Marcos, CA: Bernard Jensen Intl., 1997.

——. *Tissue Cleansing through Bowel Management.* San Marcos, CA: Bernard Jensen Intl., 1981.

Moore, Brooke Noel, and Richard Parker. *Critical Thinking.* New York, NY: McGraw-Hill Humanities, 2008.

Ha'nish, Otoman Zar-Adusht. *Distilled Water Cure.* Mrs. Clarence Gasque in Kashmir On Behalf of Mazdaznan, 1943.

Pollan, Michael. *The Omnivore's Dilemma: A Natural History of Four Meals.* New York, NY: Penguin, 2007.

Price, Weston A. *Nutrition and Physical Degeneration.* Wilkes-Barre, PA: Price-Pottenger Nutrition Foundation, 2003.

Ragnar, Peter. *How Long Do You Choose to Live?* Asheville, NC: Roaring Lion, 2001.

Wigmore, Ann. *The Blending Book.* New York, NY: Avery Trade, 1997.

INDEX

A

Absolutely Peachy, 120
Age-related macular degeneration (AMD), 28, 28n
Aging, premature, magnesium and, 29
AMD. *See* Age-related macular degeneration (AMD)
American Institute for Cancer Research, 27
American(s)
    health problems and, 5
    students, critical thinking and, 9, 9n
Anemia, 95
Anesthesia, local *vs.* general, 6–8
Ankylosing spondylitis (AS), 102–104
Anthropogenic pollution, 21
Antioxidants, 27
Appetite, green smoothies and, 112
Apple juice, 120
Apples, 120, 122, 123, 135, 137, 140, 145
Arugula, 124, 127, 145
Asch, Solomon, 9
Aspirin, headache and, 4
Atrial fibrillation, magnesium and, 29
Authority, health and, 10
Avocado, 90, 126, 127, 128, 129, 130, 131, 132, 145

B

Bananas, 118, 119, 120, 121, 123, 124, 136, 137, 138, 139, 140, 141
Basil, 127, 128, 129, 131, 132, 144, 151
Beet greens, 135, 136

Beets, 145, 150
Beet Soup, 150
Best Pudding, 138
Blackberries, 118, 140
Blackberry Strength, 118
Blender, 83, 84
Blog, 69–71
Blueberries, 124
BMC Bioinformatics, 29
Bok Choy Soup, 149
Bok choy stalks, 149
Bone repair, 15
Bones, vitamin K2 and, 31
Bowls, for produce, 83, 84
Bragg, Paul, 13
Brain function, vitamin K2 and, 31
Bread, 19–20
Breast cancer, dark green leafy vegetables and, 27
Broccoli florets, 149
Bruising, vitamin K and, 30

C

Cabbage, 150
Cabbage Salad, 147
Cancer, 27
Cantaloupe, 122
Cardiovascular disease, 26, 29
Carotenoids, foods with, 27
Carrots, 144, 145, 146, 149
Celery, 90, 127, 128, 129, 130, 132, 138, 144, 148, 152

Chard, 130, 132, 134, 137, 138
Chemicals, 21–23
Chia seeds, 135
Chronic diseases, 5, 5n, 27
Cilantro, 128, 146, 152
Cleaning supplies, natural, 83, 85
Cleansing
eliminating toxic substances during, 85
family support and, 74
healing and , 57
talking about, 70–71
Coconut, 137
Codex Alimentarius Commission, 18, 18n
Coffee, consumption of, 60, 60n
Colorectal cancer, 27
Coloring, 21
Compost bucket, 83, 85–86
Constipation, 99, 103
Consumption, of green leafy vegetables, 31
Coronary artery disease, 27, 27n
Counters, 83, 85
Cranberries, 122, 124, 136, 137, 139, 141
Cream of Broccoli Soup, 151
Cream of Sprouts, 131
Critical thinking
developing the ability of, 6–8
health and, 3–6
high-school graduates and, 9, 9n
inability to applying, 8–9
as a skill, 11
Cucumber Dill Soup, 130
Cucumbers, 119, 128, 129, 130, 131, 132, 144
Cutting boards, 83, 84

D

Daily schedule, of green smoothie retreat, 67–68
Dandelion greens, 120, 121, 132, 138
Dandelion Soup, 132
Dandelion Wine, 121
Dates, 141
Dates, Medjool, 123, 136, 139
Deficiency, illnesses and, 16
Degenerative diseases, 4
Delicious Surprise, 122
Depression, 103, 114
Detoxification, human health and, 10
"Detoxification process," 33, 35, 63–64
Detox symptoms, 35–36, 74

Diary, keeping, 69–71
Dietary fiber food, 27
Digestive problems, 98, 109
Dill, 127, 130, 131, 145, 148
Dishwashing liquids, toxicity of, 21–22

E

Ears, cupped, vitamin K and, 30
Eating, health problems and, 5
Eczema, 99
Educational materials, for healing retreat, 41–47
Emerald Applesauce, 137
Emerald Papaya, 121
Emotions, negative, green smoothies and, 109
Emptiness, following the majority and, 10
Energy
green leaves and, 26
increased, 95, 98, 99, 100–101, 103, 104, 111
Environment, restful, creating, 59–61
EPIC. See European Prospective Investigation into Cancer and Nutrition (EPIC)
Equipment, for green smoothie retreat, 83–86
European Prospective Investigation into Cancer and Nutrition (EPIC), 30
Exercise, within green smoothie retreat schedule, 67

F

Fatigue, chronic, 101–102
Fibromyalgia, magnesium and, 29
Fingers, shortened, vitamin K and, 30
Flower vase, 83, 86
Folate
deficiency in, 27, 27n
pancreatic cancer and, 27
Food additives, as defined by Codex Alimentarius Commission, 18
Foods
with carotenoids, 27
to consider purchasing, 77–78
enhancers, 21
fresh or homemade, 20
safety of, 5
in two and three hundred years ago, 4

Headache, critical thinking and, 4
Healing. *See also* Natural healing
  concentration on, 75
  of human body, 13–16
Healing retreat
  educational materials for, 41–47
  health during, 38–39
Health
  critical thinking and, 3–11
  detoxification and, 10
  green smoothies and, 108–109
  during healing retreat, 38–39
  magnesium and, 28–29
  nourishment and, 10
  primary authority on, 10
  vibrant, enjoying, 89
Health care, United States and spending
  on, 5
Health problems, 5
Heart disease, vitamin K2 and, 31
Hematomas, vitamin K and, 30
Hemorrhaging, vitamin K and, 30
Herb Garden, 130
Herbs, list of, 77
High-school graduates, critical thinking
  and, 9, 9n
Homeostasis, 16
Human body
  healing of, 13–16
  toxins and, 33–36

I

Immune system, 108–109
Immunity Strengthener, 124
Injury, healing of, 14–15
Intestinal bacterium, 31, 31n
Invitation, of people to retreat, 73–75
Iron content, in leafy vegetables, 26, 26n
Irritable bowel syndrome, 113
Italian Soup, 128

J

Judgment, 10

K

Kale, 118, 123, 129, 134, 138
Kiwi Dessert, 138
Kiwis, 119, 120, 138

Knives, 83, 84
Kombucha, 119, 120

L

Layered Green Pudding, 140–141
Lemon juice, 79
Lentils, 148
Lentils with Veggies Soup, 148
Letters from retreat participants,
  95–114
Lettuce
  butterhead, 120, 122
  green leaf, 122
  green oak, 123
  red lead, 119
  romaine, 124, 137
Lime, 119, 128, 129
Liver cancer, vitamin K and, 30
Log-book, keeping, 69–70
Loneliness, following the majority
  and, 10
Lovely Green Goodness, 123
Low-serum magnesium, 29
Lung cancer, 27

M

Macular degeneration, 27, 28, 28n
Magnesium, 27–28, 28–29
Mango, 118, 119, 120, 124, 134, 135, 136,
  137, 138
Mango Ecstasy, 134
Mango Joy, 137
McGill, Bryant, 9, 9n
Menstrual bleeding, vitamin K
  and, 30
Mental retardation, vitamin K
  and, 30
Microgreens, 146
Micro Sprout Salad, 146
Migraine disorders, magnesium and, 29
Minerals, in leafy vegetables, 26
Mint, 123, 140
Minty Delicacy, 123
Minty Lemon Desert, 136
The Miracle of Fasting (Bragg), 13
Mouth, underdevelopment of, vitamin K
  and, 30
Mushrooms, 149
Mustard leaves, 128

ABOUT THE AUTHOR

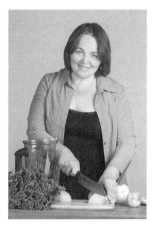 Victoria Boutenko is an acclaimed pioneer and recognized authority in the phenomenal green smoothie movement. Boutenko has appeared on Gaiam TV as well as Lifetime. Her work has been featured in Publishers Weekly, Natural Health Magazine, and the top nutrition and vegetarian publications, and her huge network of fans continues to grow. The award-winning author's popular titles include *Green For Life, Green Smoothie Revolution, Raw Family: A True Story of Awakening, 12 Steps to Raw Foods,* and *Raw Family Signature Dishes.* A raw gourmet chef, teacher, inventor, researcher, artist, and a mother of three, she teaches classes on healthy living all over the world. As a result of her teachings, millions of people are drinking green smoothies and eating raw food. Boutenko continues to travel worldwide sharing her green raw cuisine and her inspiring story of determination.